ATLAS OF
Emergency Radiology

GARY A. JOHNSON, MD

Associate Professor
Department of Emergency Medicine
SUNY Upstate Medical University
Syracuse, New York

HAL COHEN, MD

Associate Professor
Department of Radiology
SUNY Upstate Medical University
Syracuse, New York

ANDRIJ R. WOJTOWYCZ, MD

Associate Professor
Department of Radiology
SUNY Upstate Medical University
Syracuse, New York

JOHN McCABE, MD

Professor
Department of Emergency Medicine
SUNY Upstate Medical University
Syracuse, New York

ATLAS OF
Emergency
Radiology

W.B. Saunders Company
A Harcourt Health Sciences Company
PHILADELPHIA LONDON NEW YORK ST. LOUIS SYDNEY TORONTO

W.B. SAUNDERS COMPANY
A Harcourt Health Sciences Company

The Curtis Center
Independence Square West
Philadelphia, Pennsylvania 19106

Library of Congress Cataloging-in-Publication Data

Atlas of emergency radiology / Gary A. Johnson . . . [et al.].—1st ed.

p.   cm.

ISBN 0–7216–7142–X

1. Diagnosis, Radioscopic—Atlases.   2. Medical emergencies—Imaging—
Atlases.   3. Emergency medicine—Atlases.   I. Johnson, Gary A.
[DNLM: 1. Emergencies—Atlases.   2. Radiography—methods—Atlases.
3. Emergency Medical Services—methods—Atlases.   4. Wounds and
Injuries—radiography—Atlases.   WB 17 A8818 2001]

RC78.2.A85 2001   616.07′572—dc21

DNLM/DLC   00–030111

Acquisitions Editor: Stephanie Donley
Project Manager: Tina Rebane
Production Manager: Norm Stellander
Illustration Specialist: Peg Shaw

ATLAS OF EMERGENCY RADIOLOGY   ISBN 0–7216–7142–X

Printed in the United States of America.

Last digit is the print number: 9   8   7   6   5   4   3   2   1

Contributor

Louise A. Prince, MD, FACEP
Assistant Professor
The State University of New York Upstate Medical University
Syracuse, New York
Abdominal Radiography

Preface

Emergency medicine and ambulatory medical care require the mastery of a complex set of skills. These include mature and flexible interpersonal abilities, a persistent supply of compassion, multiple procedural competencies, and a working knowledge of many different databases. Patient historical, physical examination, laboratory, and radiologic data must be appropriately interpreted and synthesized into accurate and efficient diagnostic and therapeutic plans.

This text attempts to place a practical atlas of radiology in the hands of physicians who must make efficient clinical decisions. We have intentionally designed this book to be an atlas rather than a descriptive text of emergent radiology. We have also not focused on technical aspects of radiographic imaging, but rather, we aim to help the practitioner through difficult cases that involve radiologic interpretation of plain films of multiple body systems. We hope that with this text, emergency physicians and ambulatory care givers can provide a more complete and accurate diagnostic work-up of their patients.

Gary A. Johnson, MD

Hal Cohen, MD

Andrij Wojtowycz, MD

John McCabe, MD

Acknowledgments

The authors thank Diane Hartzog for her diligent and cheerful assistance in manuscript preparation.

Contents

1   Cardiothoracic Radiography 1
GARY A. JOHNSON, MD

2   Abdominal Radiography 53
LOUISE A. PRINCE, MD

3   Skull and Facial Radiography 85
GARY A. JOHNSON, MD

4   Spine Radiography 101
GARY A. JOHNSON, MD

5   Pelvic and Lower Extremity Radiography 135
GARY A. JOHNSON, MD

6   Upper Extremity Radiography 201
GARY A. JOHNSON, MD

7   Pediatric Radiography 243
GARY A. JOHNSON, MD

8   Radiography of Bone Lesions 275
GARY A. JOHNSON, MD

Index 291

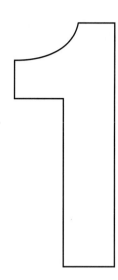

Cardiothoracic Radiography

GARY A. JOHNSON, MD

Normal Chest X-Ray Interpretation

Radiographs obtained for the chest include anteroposterior (AP), posteroanterior (PA), and lateral projections. Relatively healthy patients can stand up for routine PA and lateral views. When the patient cannot stand, the radiologist may be limited to an AP projection. Patients who are having an AP film should be sitting, if possible, but if they cannot sit, a supine radiograph may be obtained. Any routine radiograph of the chest should be obtained at the point of full inspiration (Fig. 1–1A and B). The patient should hold his or her breath, since mobile x-ray machines often require a longer exposure time and motion artifact is more easily produced.

There are many ways to read a chest radiograph. Each practitioner should develop his or her own system for reading the film and rigorously apply this system to each radiograph. Chest films in particular are rich in detail, but such details can be easily overlooked on a cursory exam. The lung fields are structures that often attract our attention initially. The only normal lung markings that are visible on radiographs are blood vessels and interlobar fissures. Blood vessels should taper out from the hilum to the periphery of the lung. Vessels are often smaller in caliber in the upper lobes than in the middle and lower lung fields. Fissures are visible if they are seen end on (i.e., in cross section). An extra fissure is observed in approximately 1% of patients, which is called an "azygos fissure" (and therefore an "azygos lobe"). A lung field should be inspected for any abnormal densities. The lung markings should extend to the periphery of the chest.

The cardiac contour and the position and size of the heart can be clearly seen on the chest film. The hilar shadows are made by lymph tissue and by pulmonary arteries and veins. The upper surface of the diaphragm is easily seen. It should be visualized from the heart shadow to the end of the costophrenic angle bilaterally. The density of the heart and the diaphragm should be similar, so that the diaphragm cannot easily be visualized below the heart. The right hemidiaphragm is often elevated more than the left, but there is much variation, both normal and abnormal. The width and depth of the costophrenic angles should be symmetric. The aortic knob should be easily identified, and the descending aorta should be visible at its left lateral contour. Age may lead to straightening or unfolding of the aorta.

The trachea and its contour should be easily visible on the frontal view. Children younger than 7 years may have a visible thymus. Young children have a large thymus that looks like a sail.

Bone structures should be examined thoroughly. Thoracic spine, sternum, ribs, clavicles, and often the scapula and proximal humerus can be examined for injuries. Bone injuries often present as "corner signs" on a chest radiograph.

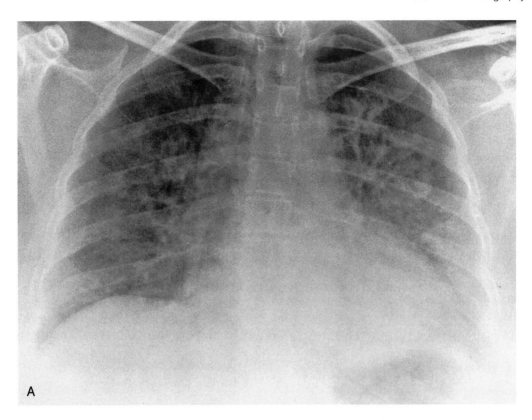

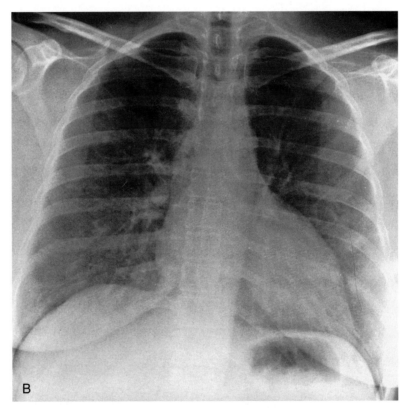

Figure 1–1
(A) *For the initial film, the patient failed to inhale deeply, and the film has the appearance of pulmonary edema.* (B) *The lungs are clear with a more optimal inspiration.*

The Heart and Vascular System

Pulmonary Edema

Congestive heart failure presents with many features across the continuum of disease associated with ventricular dysfunction. Heart failure increases pulmonary venous pressure and vascular engorgement (Fig. 1–2). As the pressure increases, fluid leaks into the interstitium. Radiographic evidence of interstitial fluid includes Kerley lines (A and B) and peribronchial cuffing. Lymphatic vessels may become visible with extreme distention. Kerley A lines extend from the hilum toward the upper and middle lung fields. Kerley B lines are horizontal, less than 2 cm long, and extend from the periphery. They are most visible at the lung bases.

Additional pulmonary vascular congestion will result in alveolar fluid and pleural effusions. Alveolar edema implies an acute process. Alveolar edema should be symmetric. It involves perihilar structures more prominently than peripheral lung fields. In extreme cases, this may give a "butterfly" appearance to the lung fields on a frontal projection. Often, lungs with baseline anatomic abnormalities exhibit an asymmetric pattern of edema that may be confused with pneumonia and atelectasis. Pulmonary edema may develop and disappear rapidly, and the time course may help to distinguish it from other infiltrates. The heart size does not change in abrupt heart failure, but chronic ventricular failure often results in cardiomegaly (Figs. 1–3, 1–4).

Noncardiogenic pulmonary edema can have many causes including toxins, high-altitude disease, neurogenic disease, and infections. In general, heart size is more likely to be normal in noncardiogenic pulmonary edema, and pulmonary vascular blood flow will probably remain normal. Air bronchograms are also unlikely to be present.

Text continued on page 10

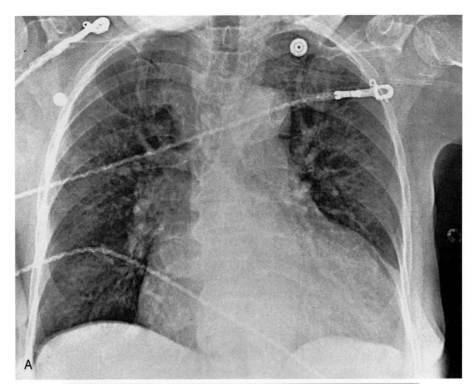

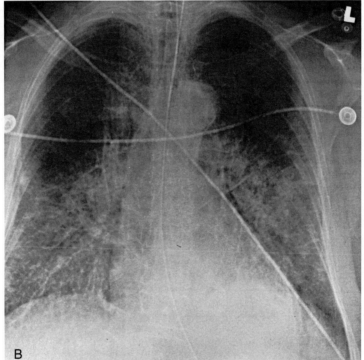

Figure 1–2

Radiographic manifestations of congestive heart failure. (A) Pulmonary venous hypertension (distended upper lobe vessels) but no interstial edema. The lack of gradation of vascular markings is often called "cephalization." Pulmonary edema can manifest radiographically in a number of ways. (B) Interstitial edema with Kerley B lines, which are best seen along the left lateral margin. They tend to be short radiopaque lines that extend to the pleura. This patient also has peribronchial thickening and some alveolar edema in the middle and lower lung fields.

Illustration continued on following page

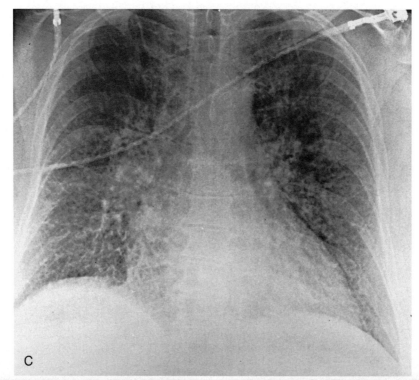

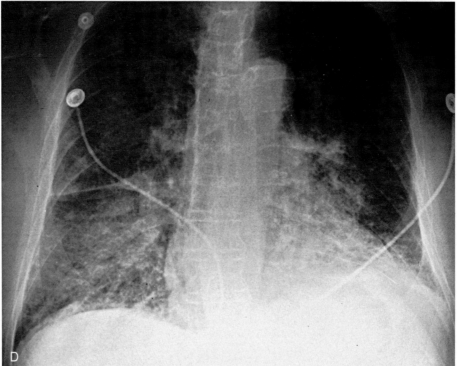

Figure 1–2 (Continued)
(C) *Interstitial pulmonary edema is manifested as prominent pulmonary vascular markings with indistinct margins and peribronchial thickening.* (D) *Alveolar and interstitial edema fluid and fluid in the minor fissure.*

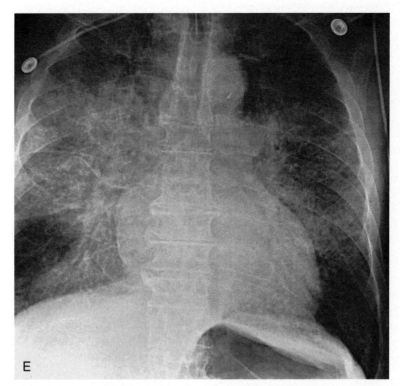

Figure 1–2 (Continued)
(E) *Alveolar pulmonary edema with a perihilar distribution.*

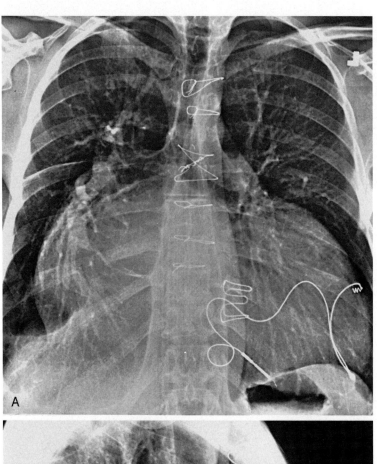

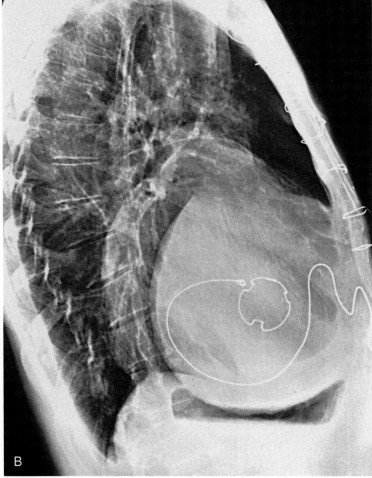

Figure 1–3
Cardiomegaly. Marked cardiomegaly is seen on both the frontal (A) and lateral (B) views of the chest. Patient also has a mitral valve prosthesis, epicardial pacing electrodes, and sternal wires. There is a small amount of fluid in the right minor fissure.

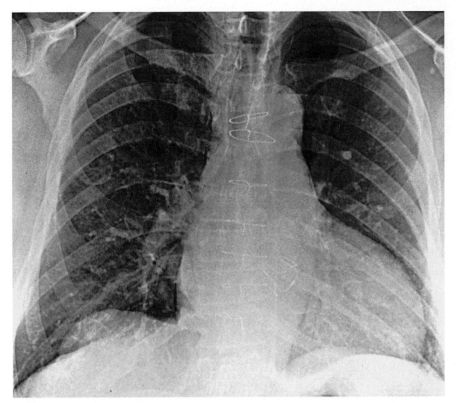

Figure 1–4
Cardiomegaly. The cardiac silhouette occupies more than 50% of the diameter of the chest on this PA view. Patient also has an artificial aortic valve.

Aneurysms

Thoracic aortic aneurysms can be true or dissecting aneurysms and can involve the ascending or descending aorta, or both. Atherosclerosis is the most common cause of aneurysms, but connective tissue disease, mycotic infections, and syphilis can also cause them. Thoracic radiographs have excellent sensitivity for demonstrating thoracic aneurysms (Figs. 1–5 through 1–7). The descending aorta and aortic knob contribute to the mediastinal silhouette. An aneurysm in these structures produces an abnormal mediastinal contour. The aortic root does not, however, contribute to the normal mediastinal shadow, and, therefore, ascending aortic aneurysms may be more difficult to diagnose.

More than 90% of thoracic aneurysms have an abnormal aortic silhouette[1]; however, aortic dilatation may be uniform and may look like an unfolded but otherwise normal aorta (Fig. 1–8). Intimal calcification may be present. If the distance between the calcified intima and the adventitia is abnormal ("calcium sign"), a dissection should be suspected. Changes in aortic width over time are most suspicious for dissection.

Abdominal aortic aneurysms are commonly calcified. They can be seen on frontal views or cross-table views of the abdomen (Fig. 1–9). When a patient's condition is stable, ultrasound and computed tomography (CT) are excellent techniques for imaging abdominal aneurysms.

Text continued on page 16

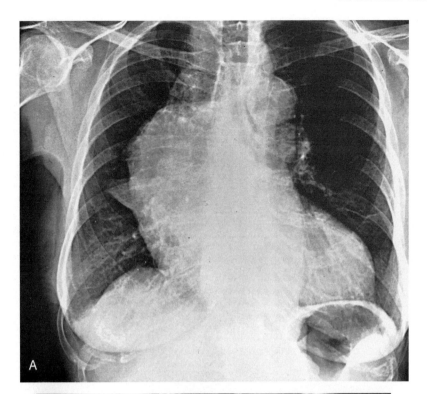

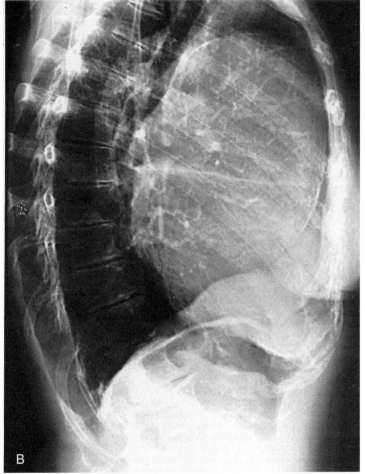

Figure 1–5
Thoracic aortic aneurysm. Ascending aorta is aneurysmal, and right middle lobe atelectasis is demonstrated.

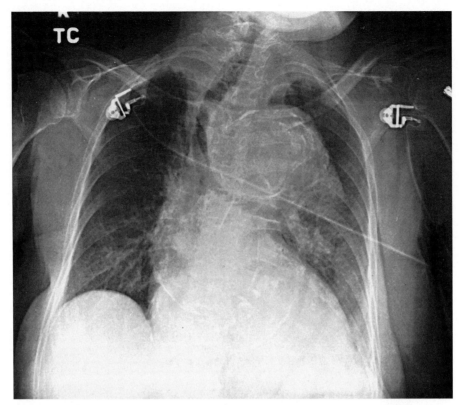

Figure 1–6
Thoracic aortic aneurysm. Intimal calcification and tracheal deviation are present.

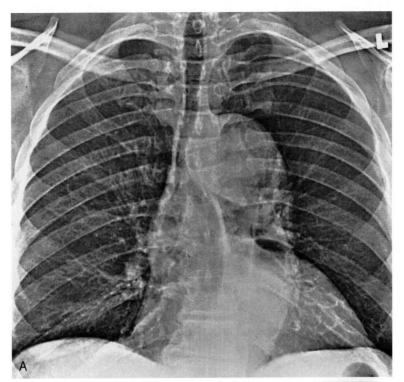

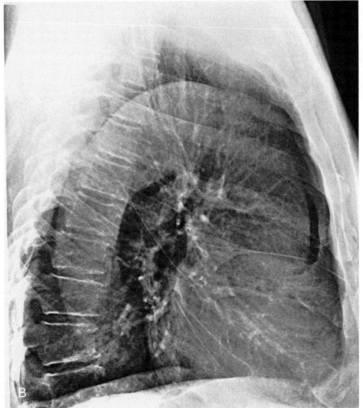

Figure 1-7
Thoracic aortic aneurysm. (A) A dilated and tortuous aorta is seen on the PA view. (B) Lateral view reveals marked dilatation of the aortic root.

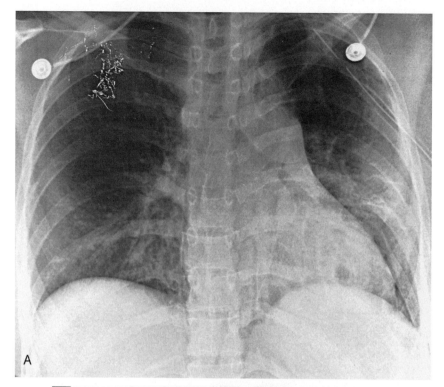

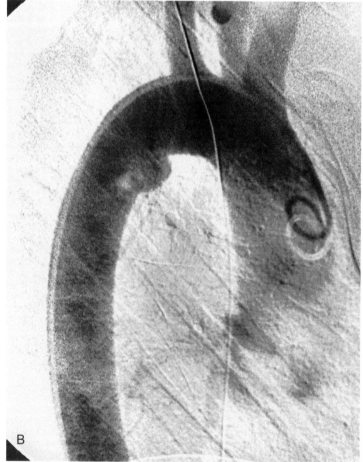

Figure 1–8
Thoracic aortic injury. (A) Original chest radiograph shows an indistinct aortic knob and descending aorta but little widening. A chest tube is on the left. (B) Angiogram demonstrates laceration of the aorta at the isthmus.

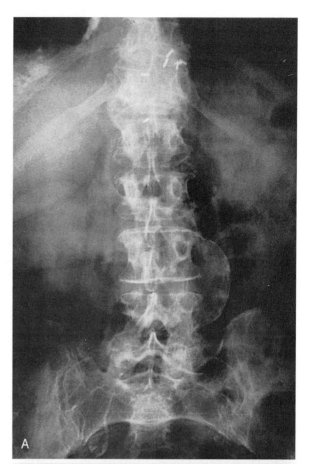

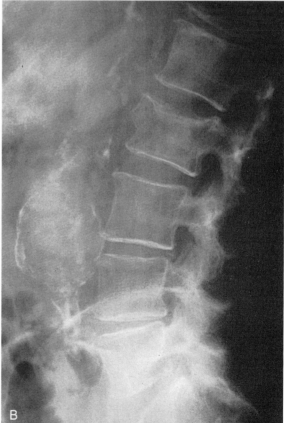

Figure 1–9
Abdominal aortic aneurysm in an elderly patient. The calcified aorta reveals a focal aneurysm that is the level of L3 and L4. This is seen on both the AP (A) and lateral (B) views. Approximately 65% of aortic aneurysms are visible on plain films.

Vascular Trauma

The chest radiograph is quite sensitive but is not specific for aortic injury. It will usually show mediastinal hematoma but not the injury itself. Many authors have sought to identify criteria that will exclude aortic injury based on plain supine radiographs of the chest,[2-5] but no single finding reliably rules it out. Mediastinal widening is the most common sign cited for suspected aortic injury. An upper limit for mediastinal width of 8.0 cm is commonly noted, although measurements have consistently been found to be insensitive. An apical pleural cap may be seen if blood has accumulated in the pleural space. This cap is more often seen in the left side of the chest. The normal paravertebral soft tissue stripe may be shifted laterally with aortic injury.

Ability to see the aortic knob and the entire descending aorta may be the most sensitive way to exclude an aortic injury (see Fig. 1–8). Two findings must be present to establish a normal film: a normal contour and no silhouetting. If possible, an erect chest radiograph should be obtained, since the patient's position frequently has a dramatic effect on the width of the mediastinum.

When aortic injury is suspected because of mechanism of injury or physical examination or x-ray findings, it can be ruled out by aortography, CT, transesophageal echocardiography, or magnetic resonance imaging (MRI),[6-10] although MRI is often difficult to do in a timely fashion. CT can reliably find mediastinal hematomas, and a normal CT study reliably excludes aortic injury. The ability to identify an aortic injury depends on the type of machine and the imaging protocol. Transesophageal echocardiography has proven to be sensitive in the hands of experienced practitioners. In many centers, aortic angiography is still considered the gold standard.

Cardiomegaly

Cardiomegaly is a common finding on chest films (see Figs. 1–3, 1–4). Cardiomegaly on radiographs does not correlate well with ventricular hypertrophy as demonstrated by echocardiogram or ECG. Cardiomegaly not known to be "old" must raise suspicion of pericardial effusion. Chest radiographs cannot rule out pericardial effusion, and, in fact, acute pericardial tamponade can occur with less than 50 ml of blood. A chronic effusion, however, will lead to enlargement of the pericardium and an enlarged cardiac silhouette.

Dextrocardia

Dextrocardia is unusual but is readily identified on a chest radiograph. Abdominal situs inversus (Fig. 1–10) may accompany dextrocardia, or intestinal rotational anatomy may be intact (Fig. 1–11).

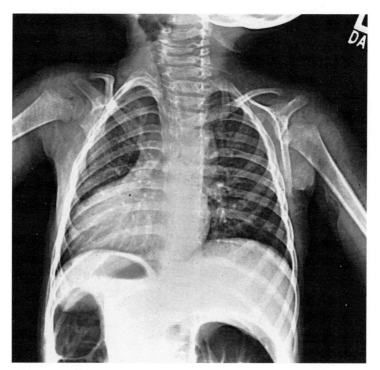

Figure 1–10
Dextrocardia and abdominal situs inversus.

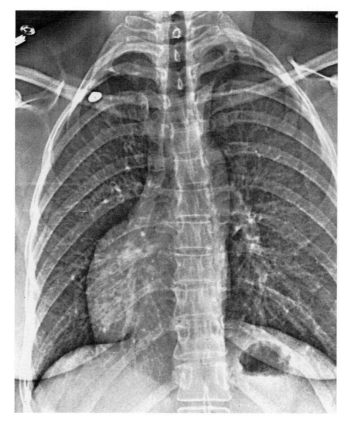

Figure 1–11
Dextrocardia with abdominal situs solitus.

Pulmonary Disease/ Pulmonary Embolus

Plain radiography generally is not helpful for demonstrating pulmonary embolus (Fig. 1–12); however, signs of infarction have been described. Hampton's hump is a pleura-based, wedge-shaped infiltrate that represents the infarcted lung parenchyma (Fig. 1–13). It is typically seen in a lower lung field. Westermark's sign is the absence of vascular markings distal to the site of an embolus with proximal dilatation of pulmonary arterial shadows. An elevated diaphragm has also been cited as an x-ray finding of pulmonary embolism.

The workup of pulmonary embolus is often a complicated matter. The ventilation-perfusion radionuclide scan is an appropriate first procedure. The PIOPED study[11] described the incidence of pulmonary embolus with high (87%), intermediate (30%), low (14%), and normal (4%) scan readings. A large number of patients have low and intermediate scans. When clinical suspicion of an embolus is high, other studies should be performed, such as lower extremity venous studies and pulmonary angiography. MRI, helical CT, and D-dimer blood assay have all been cited for possible diagnostic utility in the workup of pulmonary embolus.

Hyperinflated lung fields may be associated with obstructive airway diseases, including asthma and bronchiolitis. Children with bronchiolar inflamation (Fig. 1–14) may exhibit bronchial thickening and hyperinflation.

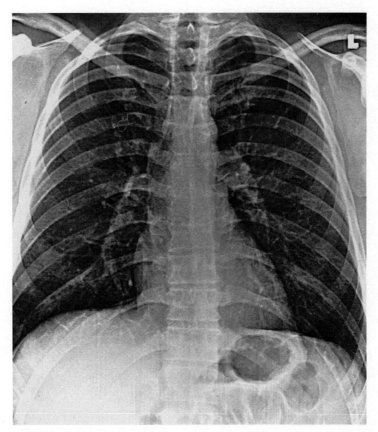

Figure 1–12
Negative chest radiograph in a patient whose ventilation-perfusion (V/Q) scan was positive.

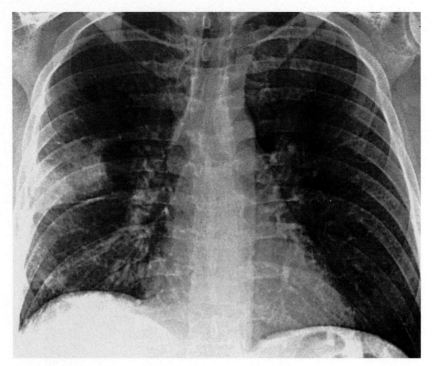

Figure 1–13
Lung infarct. The pleura-based, wedged-shaped infiltrate represents an infarct.

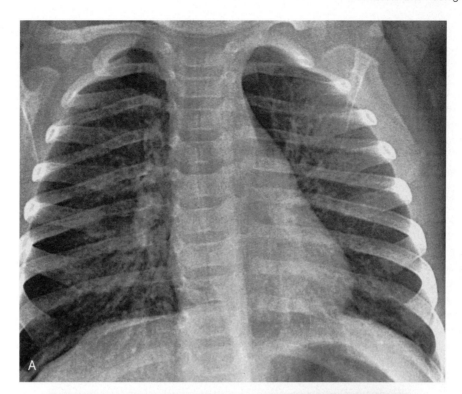

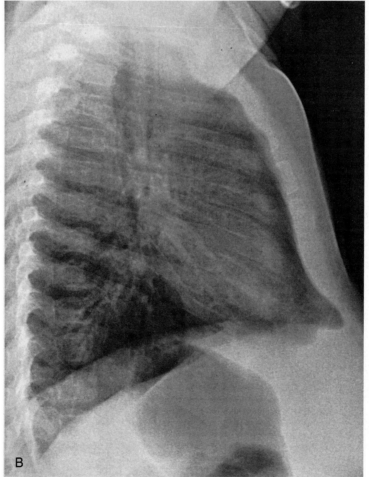

Figure 1–14
Bronchiolitis. Hyperinflation of the lungs with peribronchial thickening
is seen on both the frontal (A) and lateral (B) views.

Pweumonia

Radiographs of the chest are commonly obtained to help rule out pneumonia.[12-14] Manifestations of pneumonia on chest films are multiple. An alveolar pattern, an interstitial pattern (Figs. 1–15, 1–16), or cavitations (Fig. 1–17) may be seen. Pneumonia may be localized or diffuse. Pleural effusions and adenopathy may also be seen. Causes of pneumonia, such as a proximal obstruction from a mass or foreign body, may also be seen. Air-fluid levels may be seen with abscesses. Air-fluid levels reliably identify cavities. In the absence of fluid, the diagnosis of cavitation remains in doubt.

Alveolar infiltrates may be difficult to attribute to pneumonia, atelectasis (Fig. 1–18), tumor, or another cause. In general, a lobar infiltrate or a cavitation indicates bacterial pneumonia. Spherical infiltrates tend to indicate carcinoma, although rapid expansion may reveal the infiltrate to be a round pneumonia. Tubercular disease may be manifested as an upper lobe infiltrate or miliary nodules. Such nodules may also be seen in fungal infections.

The location of the pneumonia may be determined by the location of infiltrates as demonstrated in three dimensions by both AP and lateral films (Figs. 1–19 through 1–21). Pneumonia may be seen by silhouetting normal chest x-ray findings of similar fluid density (e.g., a right middle lobe infiltrate may silhouette out [and therefore obscure] the right heart border).

The radiographic evolution of tuberculosis includes initial consolidation of an upper lung field with hilar or mediastinal lymphadenopathy (primary complex). This process resolves and often calcifies, even without therapy. Bronchopneumonia may follow, and often it involves multiple lobes, including one or both upper lobes. Cavitation is common. Miliary spread from hematogenous infection is manifested as multiple small, well-defined nodules. Pleural effusions are common at all stages. These manifestations can clearly also appear in other illnesses. Cavitary and apical disease (Figs. 1–22, 1–23) can be bacterial or neoplastic. Effusions and pneumothorax (Figs. 1–24, 1–25) can have many causes. It is not possible to determine radiographically that tubercular disease is inactive without multiple films obtained over time.

Text continued on page 34

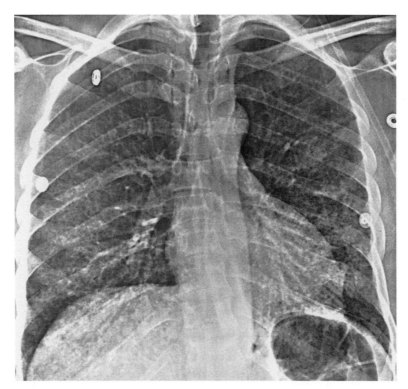

Figure 1-15
Interstitial infiltrates. The interstitial pattern is typical of Pneumocystis carinii *pneumonia.*

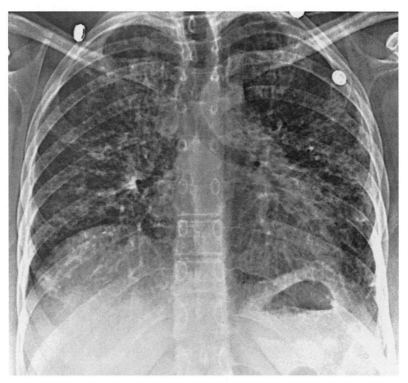

Figure 1-16
Pneumocystis carinii *pneumonia. The radiograph shows diffuse bilateral interstitial lung disease.*

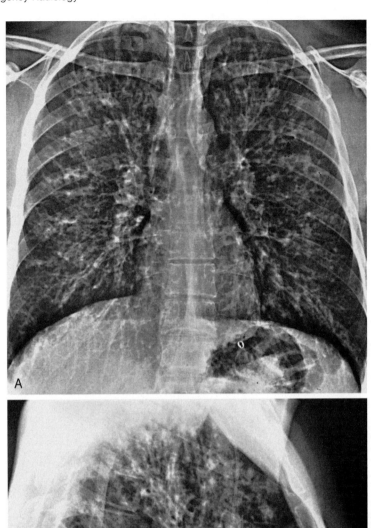

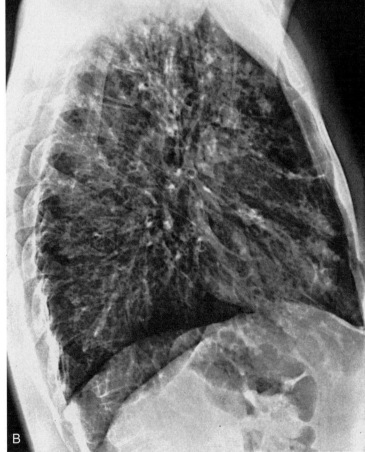

Figure 1–17
Cystic fibrosis. Diffuse interstitial pattern with peribronchial wall thickening and hyperinflation of the lungs is seen on the frontal (A) and lateral (B) views.

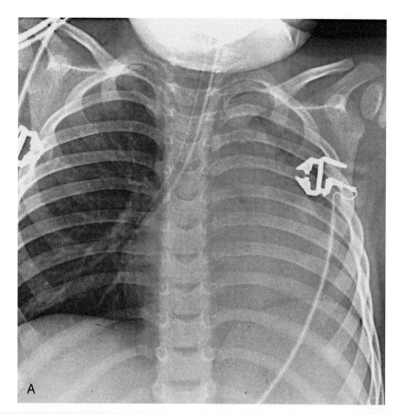

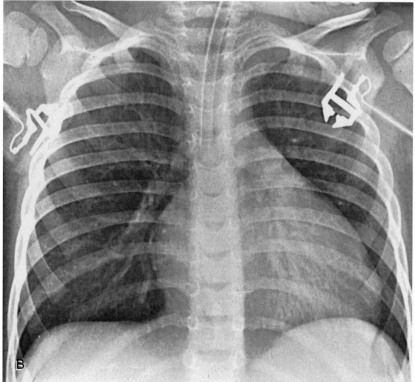

Figure 1-18

Left lung atelectasis. (A) *Opacification of the left lung field and elevation of the left diaphragm after an endotracheal tube was placed in the right mainstem bronchus. Follow-up radiograph* (B) *shows interval improvement in aeration after immediate retraction of the tube, which, however, remains too low at the level of the carina.*

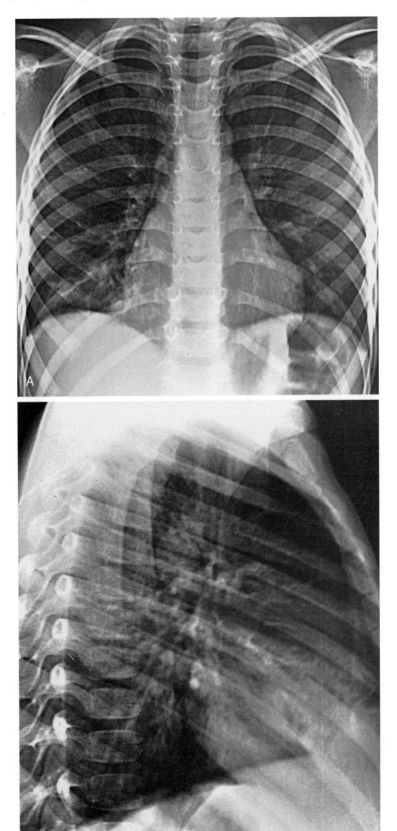

Figure 1–19

Right middle lobe pneumonia. (A) Frontal view shows increased density with poor definition of right cardiac border. (B) On the lateral film, increased density overlies the cardiac shadow.

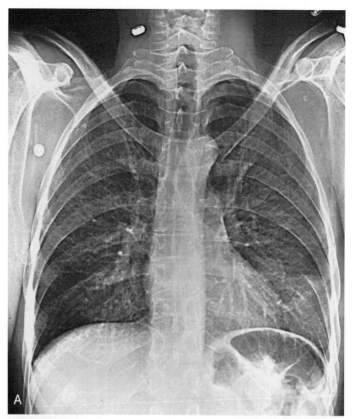

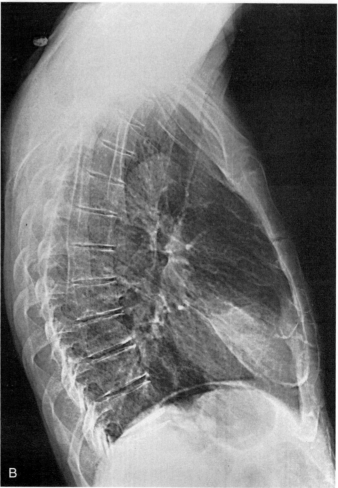

Figure 1-20
Lingular pneumonia. (A) Increased density on the frontal view partially obscures the left heart border, and increased density on the lateral exam (B) is projected over the cardiac shadow. Density on the lateral view is bordered posteriorly by the major fissure.

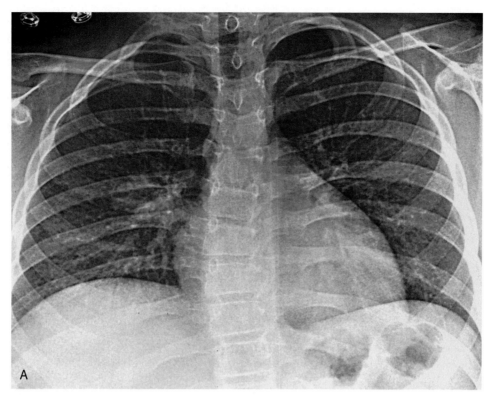

Figure 1–21
Right upper lobe pneumonia in the anterior segment. A subtle area of asymmetric increased density is visible on the frontal exam view (A) in the right perihilar region and in the retrosternal region on the lateral view (B).

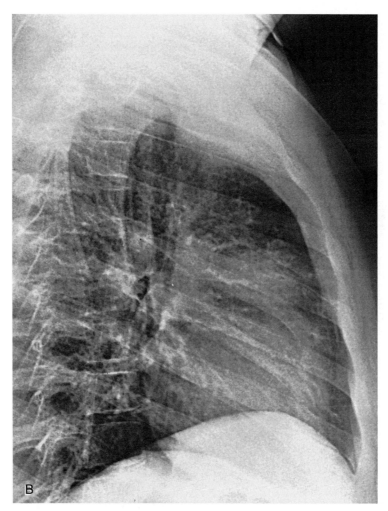

Figure 1–21 (Continued)

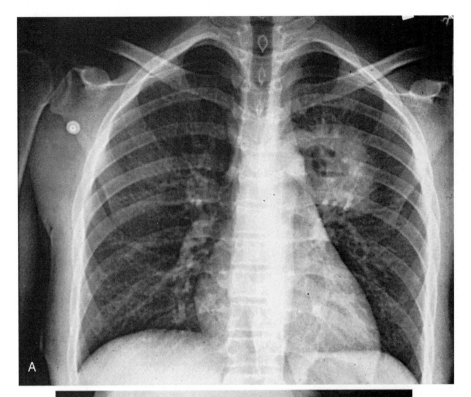

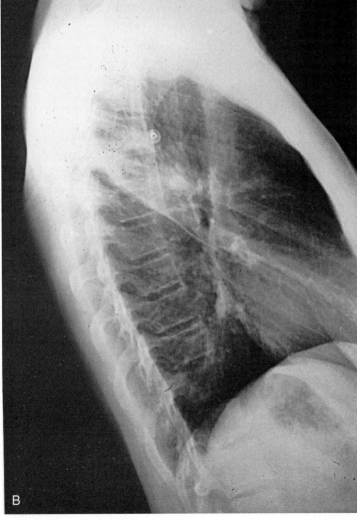

Figure 1–22
Cavitary pneumonia, posterior segment of the left upper lobe. Cavitary lesion has an air-fluid level. Differential diagnosis includes abscess, tubercular disease, and neoplasm.

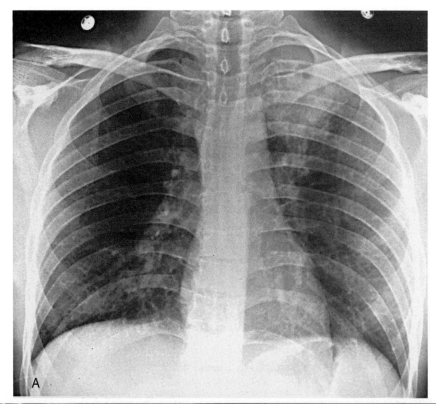

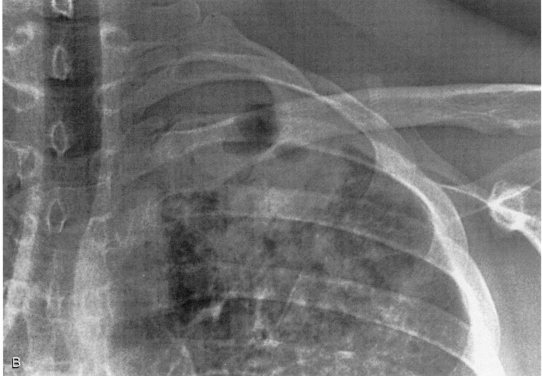

Figure 1–23
Left apical cavities in patient with methicillin-resistant Staphylococcus aureus *infection are demonstrated in frontal* (A) *and coned-down* (B) *views.*

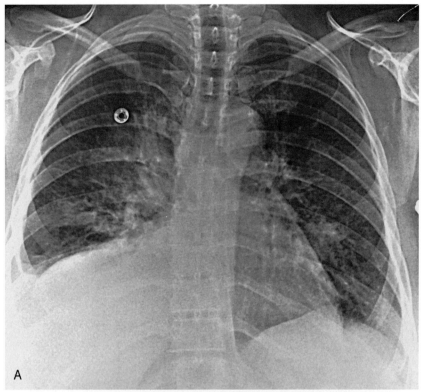

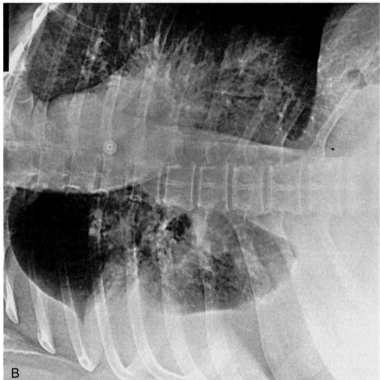

Figure 1–24

Subpulmonic effusion. (A) Frontal exam demonstrates increased density at right lung base with slight blunting of the right costophrenic angle. (B) Right lateral decubitus view shows that these findings represent a large, free-flowing pleural effusion.

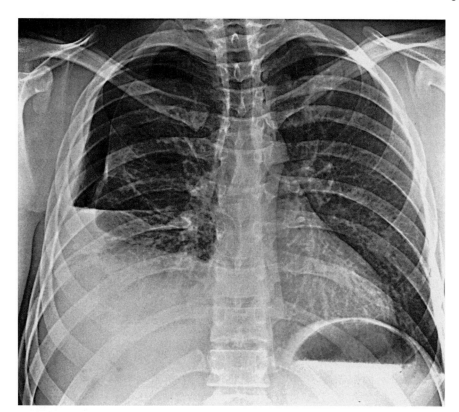

Figure 1–25
Right hydropneumothorax.

Pneumothorax and Pulmonary Trauma

Pneumothorax is common after chest trauma, whether penetrating, blunt, or even iatrogenic. Air in the pleural space violates the usual union of the visceral and parietal pleura. The most common radiographic manifestation of pneumothorax is the absence of lung markings from the visceral pleural line to the peripheral chest wall (Figs. 1–26 through 1–30). Making the diagnosis can be challenging when the pneumothorax is small. Upright expiratory radiographs may make it easier to detect. Many patients (especially trauma victims) cannot stand upright for a film. Supine radiographs may be deceiving if the air collects at the base, rather than the apex, of the lung. The pneumothorax may appear as a general decrease in density over the lung base. In a supine view, widening and deepening of the costophrenic angle—the "deep sulcus sign"— may indicate pneumothorax (Figs. 1–31, 1–32).

Radiographic methods of estimating the size of a pneumothorax have been published. The size of a pneumothorax may determine whether it is managed with a chest tube, simple aspiration, or an intrapleural catheter with a one-way valve. Most plain films underestimate the size because a plain film is a two-dimensional representation of a three-dimensional object (Fig. 1–33).

A pneumothorax that continues to collect air in the pleural space may raise intrathoracic pressure and become a tension pneumothorax. The term "tension pneumothorax" has been applied both to the clinical presentation of hemodynamic compromise and the radiographic manifestation of mediastinal shift away from the pneumothorax. A "radiographic" tension pneumothorax does not always indicate a hemodynamic tension pneumothorax.

In a trauma patient, subcutaneous emphysema may be the first sign of a lung injury that will develop into pneumothorax. Radiographically, subcutaneous emphysema is revealed by small lucencies in the soft tissue (see Fig. 1–30). A large pneumothorax may represent a tracheal bronchial rupture. Clinically, the patient has severe dyspnea, hemoptysis, and a continuous air leak after tube thoracostomy. A complete tracheobronchial tear may show that the lung is collapsed and has fallen away from the hilum ("fallen lung sign").

Air in the mediastinum may be manifested as a lucency within the mediastinal tissue, generally one that is oriented vertically in the plane of the mediastinum (Fig. 1–34). Air between the diaphragm and the pericardium allows visualization of the entire diaphragm. Air may also be seen in the pericardium or in the soft tissues of the neck.

Fluid in the pleural space has several manifestations. It can be subpulmonic (Fig. 1–24) or be accompanied by pneumothorax (Fig. 1–25). Fluid within a fissure can appear to be a mass (Fig. 1–35). Disruption of the pulmonary parenchyma may form a pulmonary laceration. This often is accompanied by a local hematoma. Traumatic lung cysts are also common and they persist after the hematoma resolves (Figs. 1–36 through 1–39). Radiographs show patchy infiltrates and a cystic mass. These infiltrates may contain air-fluid levels.

Blunt abdominal or blunt chest trauma often causes a diaphragmatic rupture, as may a penetrating injury to the lower chest or upper abdomen. Small diaphragmatic tears or ruptures may be radiographically inapparent (Figs. 1–40 through 1–42). Other radiographic findings may suggest a diaphragmatic injury by revealing an elevated hemidiaphragm and an indistinct diaphragmatic shadow. A more obvious diaphragmatic rupture may reveal abdominal contents, such as bowel gas, in the chest. Atelectasis or pleural effusion may make this diagnosis difficult by plain radiography. When further workup is necessary, CT or barium swallow studies are appropriate.

Text continued on page 46

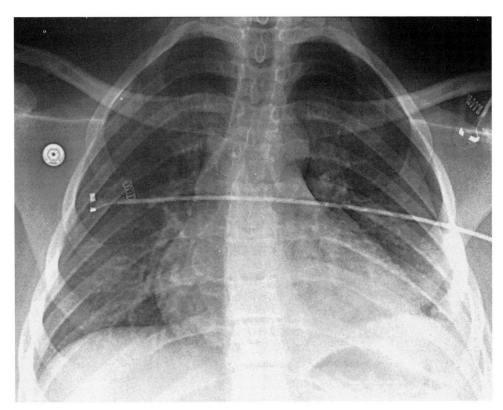

Figure 1–26
Left pneumothorax.

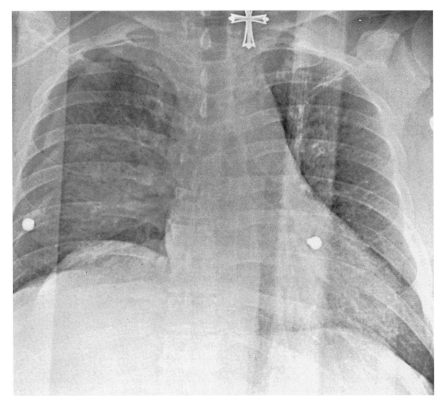

Figure 1–27
Right pneumothorax. Intrapleural air is visible at the lateral margin of the right lung.

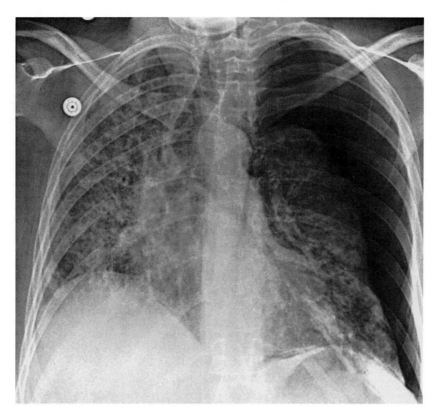

Figure 1–28
Left tension pneumothorax in patient with Pneumocystis carinii *pneumonia has shifted mediastinal structures to the right.*

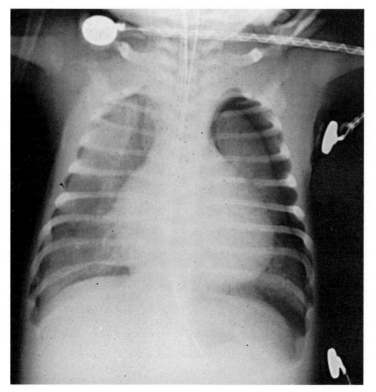

Figure 1–29
Bilateral pneumothorax. This patient has broncho-pulmonary dysplasia, which produces an image called "ground-glass lungs." A pneumothorax is clearly visible along the entire left lateral margin of the chest. A smaller pneumothorax is also visible on the right base.

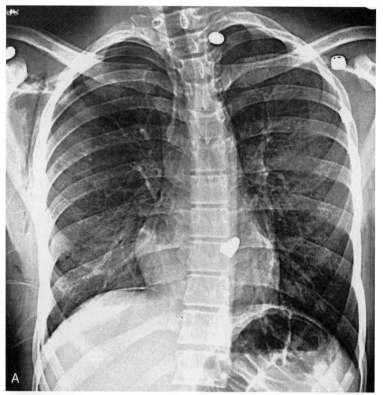

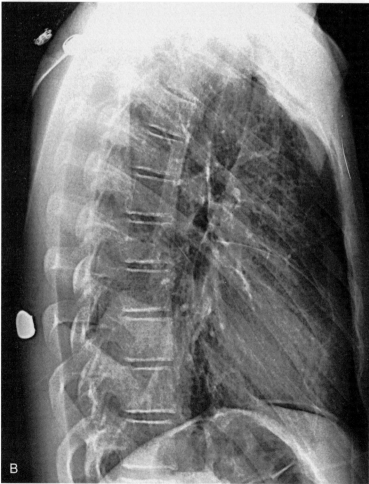

Figure 1–30

Multiple findings in a trauma patient in frontal (A) and lateral (B) views. A bullet is lodged in subcutaneous tissues posterior to and to the left of the thoracic spine. Free air is visible in the abdomen. Right pneumothorax, right lower lung contusion, and subcutaneous air in the right lateral chest wall are also demonstrated.

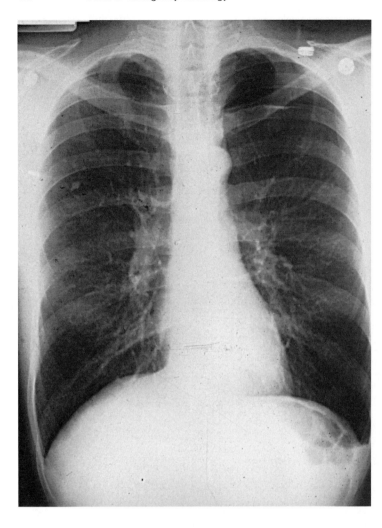

Figure 1–31
Left apical pneumothorax with deep sulcus sign. The left costopulmonary angle is blunted and widened. This deep sulcus sign is often associated with pneumothorax in patients who cannot stand for chest radiography. Eleven ribs are visible with inspiration, a finding consistent with hyperinflation.

Figure 1–32
This patient has a pneumothorax that is manifested principally at the left base. This produces a deep sulcus sign. The costophrenic angle is wider, and in this case farther inferior.

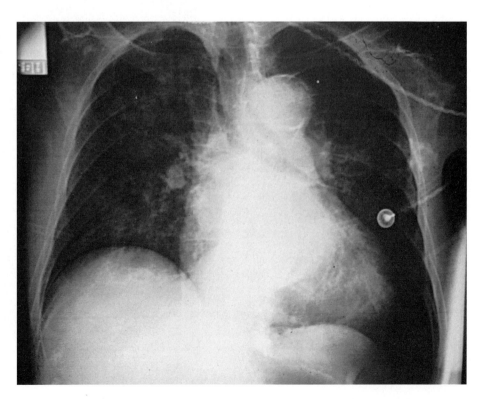

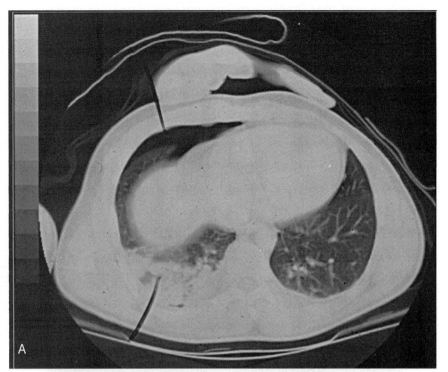

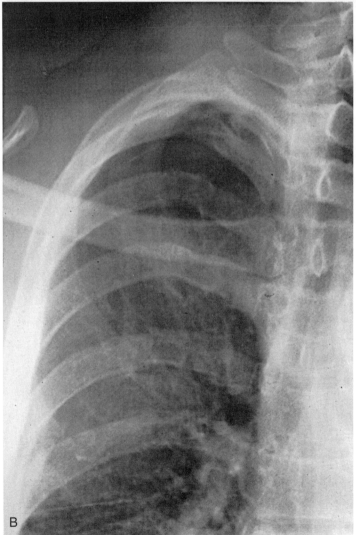

Figure 1–33

Plain radiography affords a gross estimate of the size of a pneumothorax. Many pneumothoraces, like the one seen on CT (A), are barely visible or are invisible on plain film (B). This is especially problematic in supine patients.

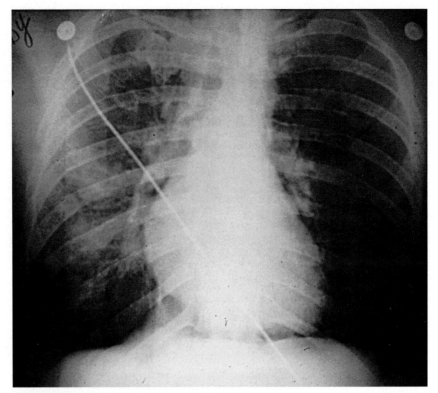

Figure 1–34
*Pneumomediastinum. The pneumomediastinum has lifted the heart off the dia-
phragm (air extends between the pericardium and the diaphragm). This allows
for visualization of the entire diaphragm and has been called the "continuous
diaphragm" sign.*

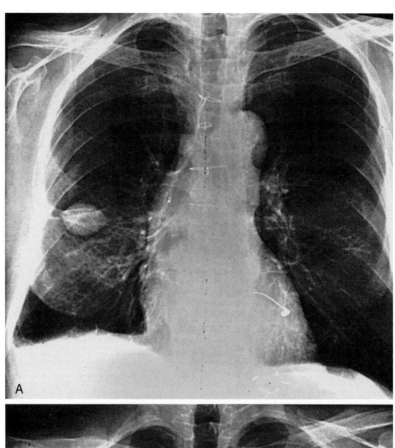

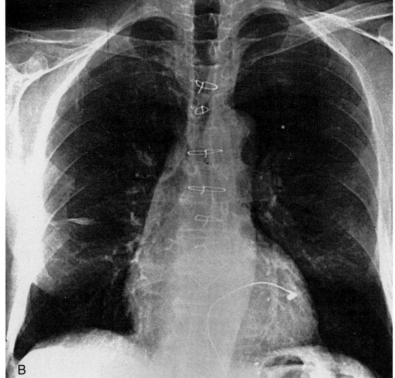

Figure 1–35

Pseudotumor. (A) *Fluid in minor fissure causes an oval opacification in the region of the minor fissure. Also, mild blunting of the right costophrenic angle is consistent with a small pleural effusion.* (B) *On follow-up exam, a decrease in the amount of fluid in the minor fissure and right costophrenic angle is seen.*

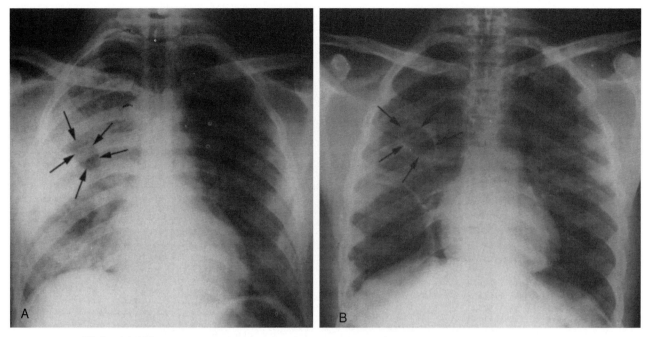

Figure 1–36

(A) *A 3-cm rounded radiolucency* (arrows) *is demonstrated within a large pulmonary contusion that was incurred during a motor vehicle accident.* (B) *A posteroanterior film taken after resolution of the pulmonary contusion demonstrates a simple cavity* (arrows)*; this is the residual pulmonary laceration. (Redman HC, Purdy PO, Miller GL, Rollins NK: Emergency Radiology. Philadelphia: WB Saunders, 1993.)*

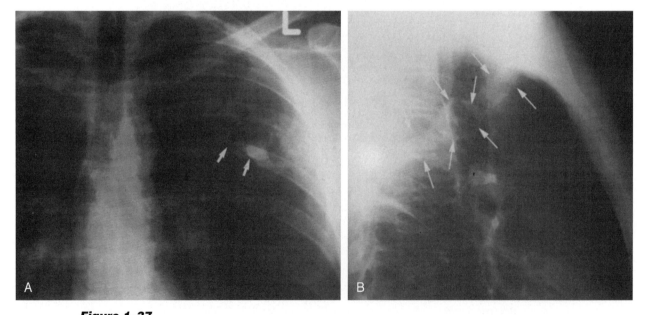

Figure 1–37

A pulmonary laceration was produced by a bullet as it passed obliquely through the left side of the chest. (A) *PA film demonstrates both a lucent lesion and a small area of consolidation* (arrows)*.* (B) *The lateral view demonstrates the tubular nature of the laceration even more clearly* (arrows)*. (Redman HC, Purdy PO, Miller GL, Rollins NK: Emergency Radiology. Philadelphia, WB Saunders, 1993.)*

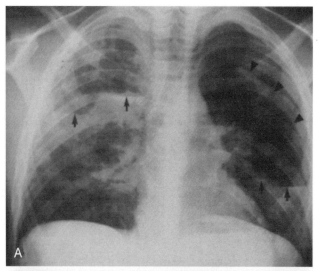

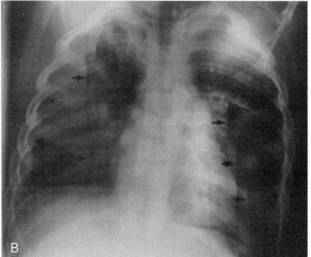

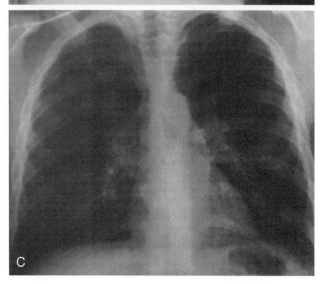

Figure 1–38

Extensive pulmonary contusion and laceration. (A) Extensive bilateral infiltrates with multiple air-fluid levels (arrows) in a 10-year-old boy following a motor vehicle accident. Note also the large left pneumothorax (arrowheads). (B) A right lateral decubitus film shows the numerous air-fluid levels to even better advantage (arrows). A small right pleural effusion is present (arrowhead). (C) A follow-up PA film obtained 3 weeks after injury shows almost complete resolution of the extensive bilateral parenchymal injury. (Redman HC, Purdy PO, Miller GL, Rollins NK: Emergency Radiology. Philadelphia, WB Saunders, 1993.)

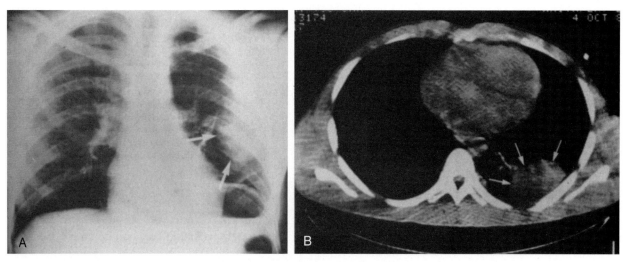

Figure 1–39

Posttraumatic pulmonary hematoma. (A) PA film obtained 3 days after a motor vehicle accident demonstrates a large mass laterally near the base of the left lung (arrows). (B) The mass is also well seen on this CT scan (arrows). The appearance on CT is typical of a hematoma that resolved completely after a few months. (Redman HC, Purdy PO, Miller GL, Rollins NK: Emergency Radiology. Philadelphia, WB Saunders, 1993.)

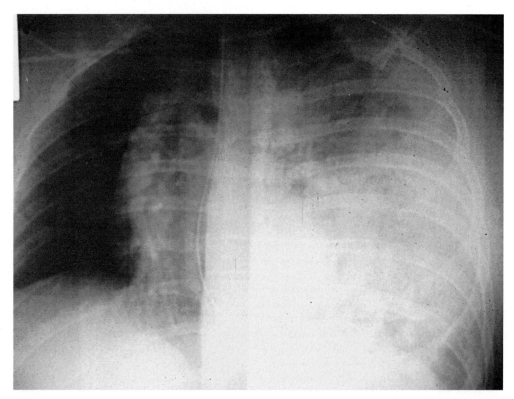

Figure 1–40

Diaphragm rupture. Peritoneal contents are herniated into the left chest. Haustral markings are visible in the left chest.

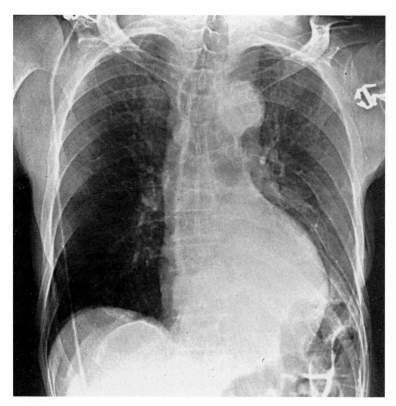

Figure 1–41
Rupture of the left hemidiaphragm. The left hemidiaphragm is not visualized, and bowel is seen in the left chest.

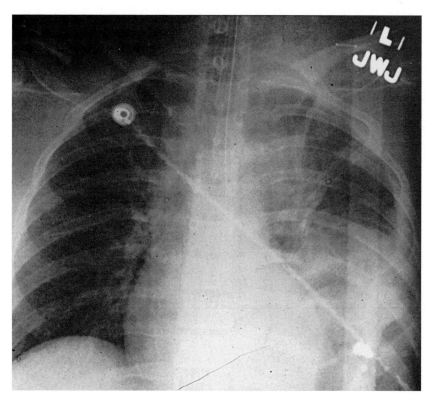

Figure 1–42
Diaphragmatic rupture.

Sternal Fracture

Sternal fracture may be difficult to see on routine chest radiograph views. A coned-down lateral may be helpful (Fig. 1–43). Sternal views with an oblique frontal approach may also show the fracture. It is possible to disrupt one table of the sternal wall, leaving the rest intact (similar to a skull injury).

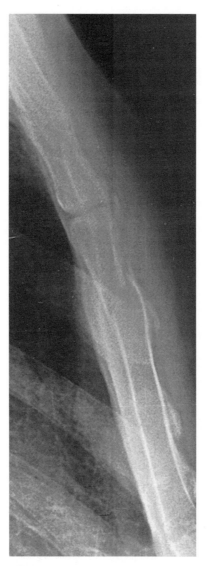

Figure 1–43
Sternal fracture. Lateral view of the sternum shows a fracture of the anterior and posterior cortices.

Lung Masses and Anatomic Variants

Pulmonary masses may be hilar (Fig. 1–44) or intraparenchymal (Figs. 1–45, 1–46). Lymphadenopathy, tumors, granulomas, or developmental variants may account for mass lesions.

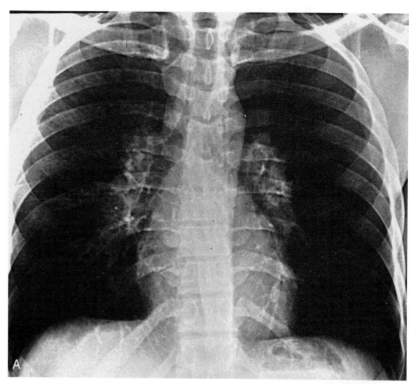

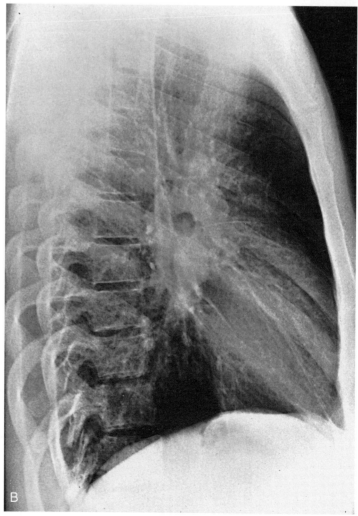

Figure 1–44

Sarcoidosis. Symmetric bilateral hilar enlarge-
ment secondary to hilar adenopathy is seen on
frontal (A) and lateral (B) views. Right peritra-
cheal adenopathy is also present.

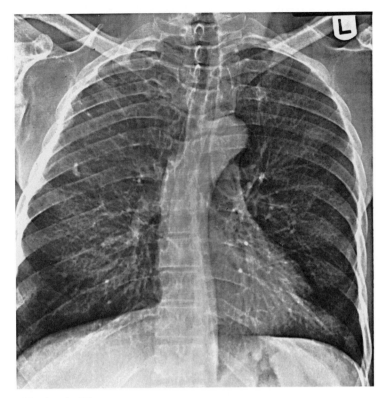

Figure 1–45
Right midlung granuloma.

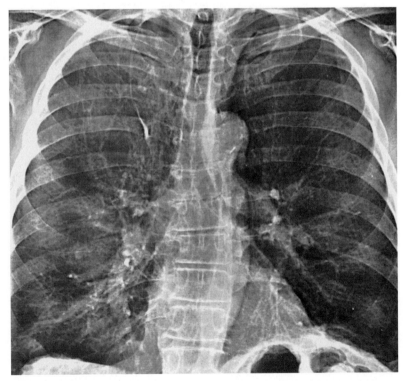

Figure 1–46
Azygous lobe. This developmental variant, an anomalous fissure, may be confused with a cavitary lesion.

REFERENCES

1. Petre R, Von Segresser LK: Aortic dissection. Lancet 1997;349(9063):1461–1464.

2. Seltzer SE, D'Orsi C, Kirshner R, et al: Traumatic aortic rupture: Plain radiographic findings. AJR 1981;137:1011–1014.

3. Simeone JF, Deren MM, Cagle F: The value of the left apical cap in the diagnosis of aortic rupture. Radiology 1981;139:35–37.

4. Mirvis SE, Bidwell JK, Buddemeyer EU: Value of chest radiography in excluding traumatic aortic rupture. Radiology 1987;163:487–493.

5. White CS, Mirvis SE: Pictorial review: Imaging of traumatic aortic injury. Clin Radiol 1995;50:281–287.

6. Mirvis SE, Shanmuganathan K, Miller BH, et al: Traumatic aortic injury: Diagnosis with contrast-enhanced thoracic CT—five-year experience at a major trauma center. Radiology 1996;200(2):413–422.

7. Ahrar K, Smith DC, Bansal RC, et al: Angiography in blunt thoracic aortic injury. J Trauma 1997;42(4):665–669.

8. Driscoll PA, Hyde JA, Curzon I, et al: Traumatic disruption of the thoracic aorta: A rational approach to imaging. Injury 1997;27(10):679–685.

9. Sarasin FP, Louis-Simonet M, Gaspoz JM, et al: Detecting acute thoracic aortic dissection in the emergency department: Time constraints and choice of the optimal diagnostic test. Ann Emerg Med 1996;28(3):278–288.

10. Pretre R, Chilcott M: Current concepts: Blunt trauma to the heart and great vessels. N Engl J Med 1997;336(9):626–632.

11. PIOPED: Value of the ventilation/perfusion scan in acute pulmonary embolism. JAMA 1990;263(20):2753–2759.

12. Brown PD, Lerner SA: Community-acquired pneumonia. Lancet 1998;352(9136):1295–1302.

13. Bartlett JG, Mundy LM: Current concepts: Community-acquired pneumonia. N Engl J Med 1995;333(24):1618–1624.

14. Jadavji T, Law B, Lebel M, et al: A practical guide for the diagnosis and treatment of pediatric pneumonia. Can Med Assoc J 1997;156(Suppl 5):703S–711S.

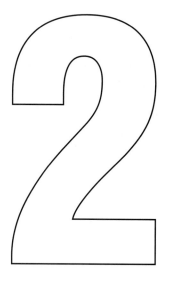

Abdominal
Radiography

LOUISE A. PRINCE, MD

The clinician evaluating a patient with abdominal pain should have a clear understanding of which diagnostic tests are likely to be of help for a specific clinical presentation and of the limitations of the tests being ordered. For the majority of patients who present with abdominal pain, the diagnosis is elucidated by history and physical examination alone. Plain abdominal radiography can help to verify diagnostic suspicions. Before a clinician orders plain abdominal radiographs, she should step back and consider whether these studies are likely to show what is being sought.

Many authors have investigated the utility of abdominal radiographs. Eisenberg and coworkers[1] noted that reserving such studies for cases of "moderate or severe" abdominal tenderness or a high suspicion of bowel obstruction, calculi, or ischemia would eliminate 54% of examinations without limiting the number of "significant" findings. Campbell and Gunn[2] found that radiographic findings were often insignificant for the investigation of suspected appendicitis, urinary tract infection, and nonspecific abdominal pain. Rothrock and colleagues[3] investigated radiographs of children and noted that limiting studies to patients who have had surgery or who have a suspected foreign body, abnormal bowel sounds, abdominal distention, or peritoneal signs identified all patients with radiographs that were diagnostic for a major disease. With their system, 48% of studies could be eliminated.

Plain Radiographs

The supine abdominal film is usually the first to be performed. It is a view of the abdomen from the diaphragm to the symphysis pubis. Bony structures such as the spine, lower ribs, and portions of the pelvis are visible. Soft tissues such as the edge of the psoas muscle and margins of the liver, spleen, and kidneys may be identified. A heavily calcified aorta may be seen, as may nephrolithiasis or cholelithiasis. Visualizing suspicious calcifications is not truly diagnostic of nephrolithiasis, nor is visualization of biliary stones helpful in diagnosing cholecystitis or biliary obstruction. Bowel gas patterns suggestive of either cecal or sigmoid volvulus are also seen on the supine film. Occasionally, evidence of mass effect may be seen as well with lesions such as large tumors, pelvic hematomas, and organomegaly. Foreign bodies are readily identified. Bowel wall edema may be seen, and its appearance is commonly referred to as "thumbprinting." Air in the bowel wall, pneumatosis intestinalis, can be seen as well.

Positional radiographs are made after the supine film. These include upright and/or lateral decubitus films. These views help elucidate bowel gas patterns. Dilatation of small or large bowel may be visualized, as may air-fluid levels. Patterns of bowel dilatation and air-fluid levels are diagnostic of bowel obstruction. Likewise, areas of small bowel dilatation and air-fluid levels may indicate localized ileus that represents a reaction to a nearby infectious or inflammatory process. These areas of ileus are called "sentinel loops" and may be seen in pancreatitis, appendicitis, and cholecystitis. The upright film may show air beneath the diaphragm, which is indicative of a perforated hollow viscus. Lateral decubitus films may also show free air along the superior edge of the abdomen. Upright chest radiographs are superior to abdominal films for demonstrating air beneath the diaphragm. The usefulness of a three-film study (supine abdomen, upright abdomen, and upright chest) has been questioned. Mirvis and associates[4] found that 98% of abnormalities in emergency department patients could be seen on the supine abdominal film and the erect chest film.

One additional abdominal radiograph is occasionally warranted—the cross-table lateral view. This film may demonstrate an abdominal aortic aneurysm if the vessel is heavily calcified. It can help to verify clinical suspicions when a patient is too ill to undergo imaging studies that might be more discriminating, but it is not sensitive. A cross-table view has also been described for visualizing early pneumoperitoneum in children.[5]

Clinical Situations

Plain radiographs are extremely useful for confirming diagnoses that fall into these categories: small bowel obstruction, ileus, cecal and sigmoid volvulus, colonic obstruction, and possibly intussusception leading to obstruction. Proximal obstruction, such as gastric outlet obstruction or gastric atony (Fig. 2–1), may be associated with minimal findings on radiographs. Abnormal air collections are unusual. Solid gastric contents may be visible. Distended loops of small bowel are identified by evidence of plicae circulares or valvulae conniventes (which look like stacks of coins) that completely cross the diameter of the bowel (Fig. 2–2). Large bowel is identified by haustra that do not completely cross the diameter of the bowel. Air-fluid levels indicate cessation of peristalsis, causing stagnation of fluid and air. These often have a stepladder pattern when they are located in the small bowel. For air to enter the small bowel, the ileocecal valve must be incompetent, allowing air to pass in retrograde fashion. If the ileocecal valve is competent, the small bowel may be completely filled with fluid and have the appearance of ground glass (ascites also has this appearance). In patients with a competent ileocecal valve, colonic obstruction leads to distention of the cecum. Distention of the cecum past 9 cm increases the danger of perforation. Intussusception may give the appearance of large bowel obstruction.

Small amounts of intraluminal gas without a clear-cut obstruction has been termed a "nonspecific abdominal gas pattern." Patel and Lauber[6] found that radiologists and referring physicians had significant differences in interpretation of these words when used in an official reading of abdominal radiographs. They recommended that the term "nonspecific abdominal gas pattern" be abandoned.

Adynamic or paralytic ileus occurs when peristalsis ceases as a result of local infection or inflammation such as pancreatitis, appendicitis, or generalized illness such as myxedema or congestive heart failure. There may be localized or generalized distention of small and large bowel with air-fluid levels (Fig. 2–3). The air-fluid levels may not be as prominent as in mechanical obstruction.

Sigmoid volvulus appears as a distended loop of colon emerging from the pelvis. The enlarged bowel twists. The area of rotation has the appearance of a bird's beak, and air-fluid levels may be present within the volvulus. Cecal volvulus is likewise twisting of the cecum on its axis. Typically, the dilated loop is located in the epigastrium or left upper quadrant (Fig. 2–4). It may have a kidney bean appearance.

Midgut volvulus may present in neonates as mechanical obstruction. Air is visible only in the proximal gut (Fig. 2–5).

Constipation is often considered when a patient who seems otherwise well complains of having no bowel movements. A plain radiograph of the abdomen demonstrates large amounts of stool in the colon, verifying the diagnosis (Fig. 2–6). Intestinal obstruction can likewise be ruled out.

Bowel wall findings are nonspecific. Bowel wall edema or hemorrhage may be seen in the setting of mesenteric ischemia. This may give the appearance of thumbprinting within the bowel wall. Pneumatosis intestinalis (Figs. 2–7, 2–8) is a rare finding of air within the wall of the intestine associated with diseases such as necrotizing enterocolitis and chronic obstructive pulmonary disease, leading to dissection of air through the mediastinum down into the peritoneum.

Herniated bowel may present as air in unusual locations or as a mass. Inguinal herniated bowel may be manifested as intraluminal gas seen outside the abdominal cavity (Fig. 2–9). Hiatal hernia may move intrathoracic structures (Fig. 2–10) or may be associated with intraluminal gas in the chest.

Text continued on page 68

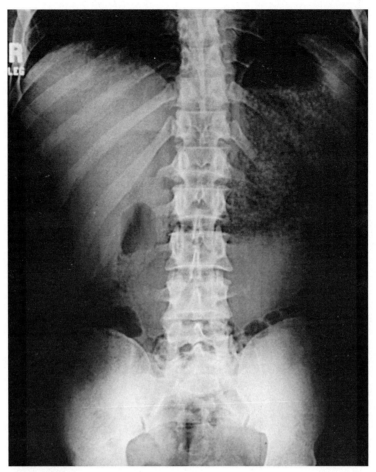

Figure 2–1
Dilated stomach with speckled appearance, which is consistent with bezoar or gastric atony.

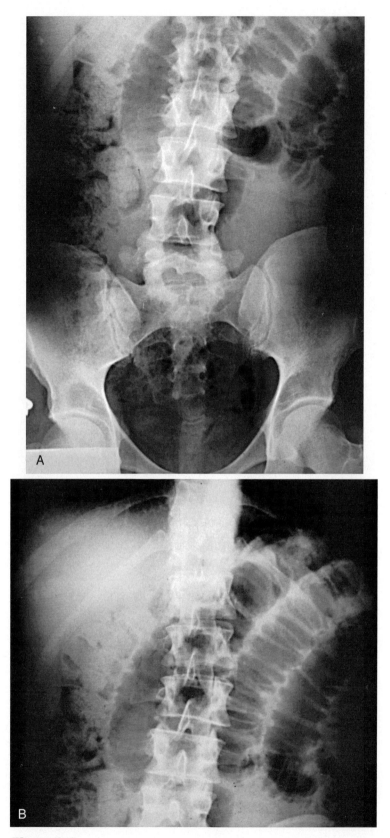

Figure 2–2

Dilatation of small bowel. (A, B) Plicae circulares help to identify the bowel as small bowel. In comparison, the colon is not dilated and contains stool. This gas pattern suggests a partial small bowel obstruction or focal small bowel ileus.

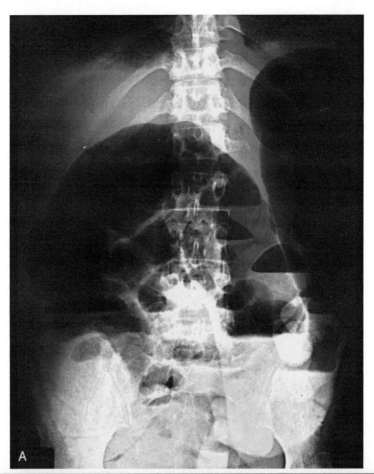

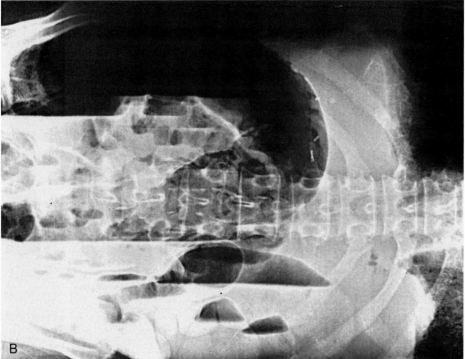

Figure 2–3
Ileus. (A) Upright and (B) decubitus views reveal diffusely distended bowel, both large and small, with air-fluid levels.

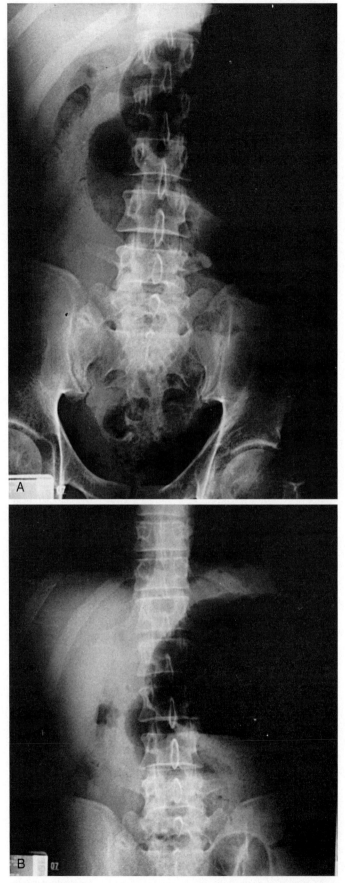

Figure 2–4
Cecal volvulus. (A, B) Plain radiographs show a very dilated loop of bowel in the left upper quadrant.

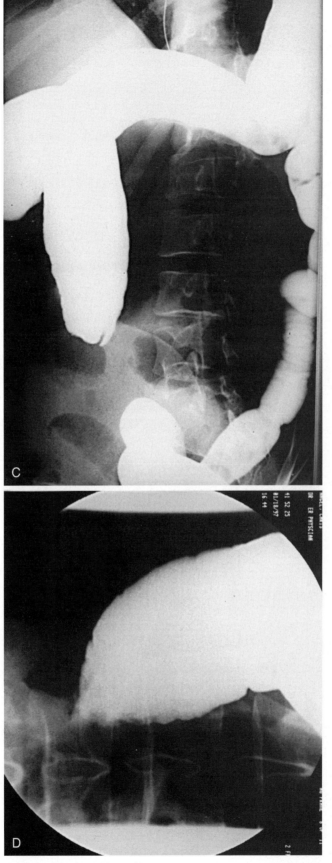

Figure 2–4 (Continued)
(C, D) *Barium enema studies reveal "bird's beak" appearance typical of cecal volvulus.*

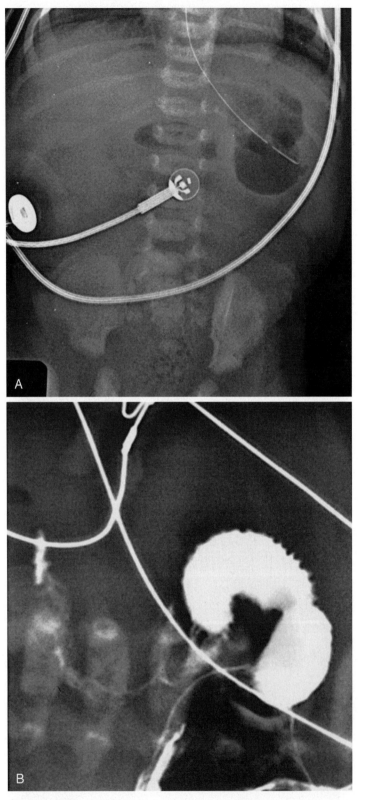

Figure 2–5
Midgut volvulus. (A) On scout film, air is demonstrated in stomach and proximal duodenum. There is a paucity of air distally. Nasogastric tube in stomach. (B, C) Upper gastrointestinal series. Tapering of the third portion of duodenum. Contrast does not extend to the left of midline on the frontal view but instead extends into the right lower quadrant in a "corkscrew" pattern.

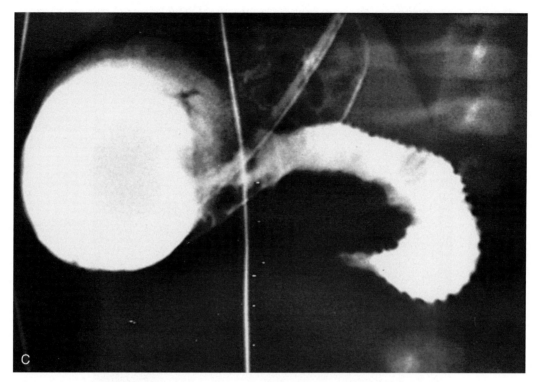

Figure 2–5 (Continued)

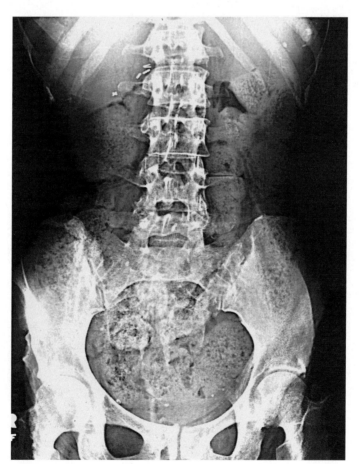

Figure 2–6
Constipation. Note large volume of stool throughout the entire colon.

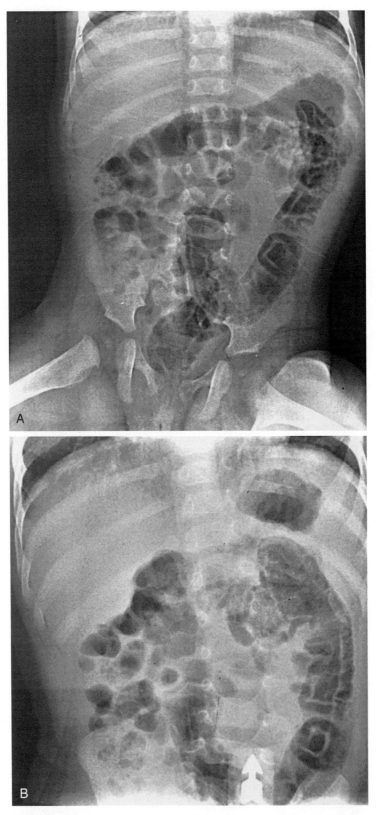

Figure 2–7
Pneumatosis intestinalis. (A) *Air is visible in the bowel wall (colon) of a child.* (B) *Upright view shows no free air under the diaphragm.*

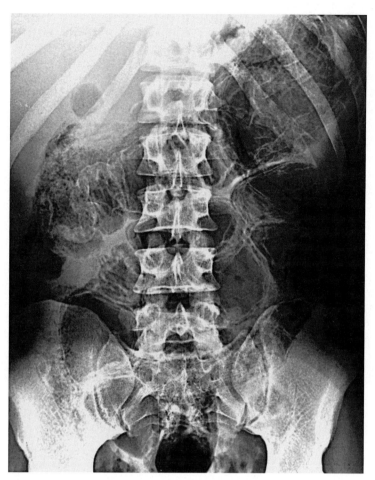

Figure 2–8
Pneumatosis intestinalis. Air is present in the intestinal wall.

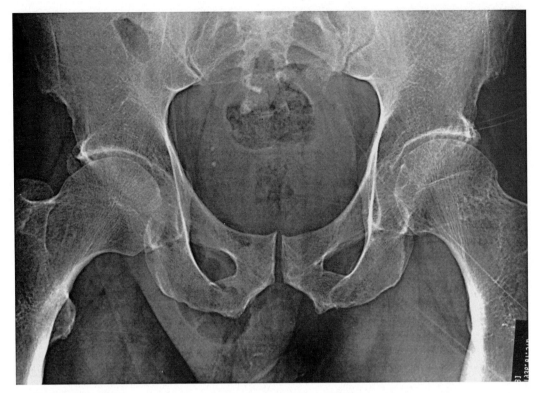

Figure 2–9
Right inguinal hernia. Bowel with air is visible in the inguinal canal and overlying the right pubic ramus.

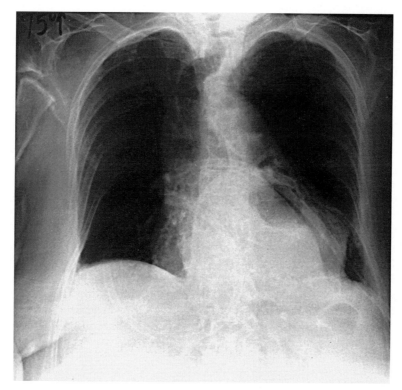

Figure 2-10

Large hiatal hernia: Note the retrocardiac soft tissue density, which also contains air. Buckling of the trachea is due to ectasia of the mediastinal vasculature.

Radiopaque Structures

Approximately 80% of renal calculi and 20% of biliary calculi (Fig. 2–11) are radiopaque. A plain abdominal radiograph may demonstrate what appears to be nephrolithiasis owing to the position of the calcified stone, but the gold standard for identifying nephrolithiasis and ureteral calculi that are causing obstruction is the intravenous pyelogram or CT. Plain abdominal radiographs are not indicated for diagnosing cholelithiasis. Ultrasound and hepatobiliary iminodiacetic acid (HIDA) scanning have more diagnostic utility.

Abnormal gallbladder wall calcification may indicate biliary cancer (Fig. 2–12). Air and air-fluid collections in the gallbladder indicate emphysematous cholecystitis (Fig. 2–13).

The aorta may be identified on plain radiographs if it is heavily calcified. On rare occasions, in an extremely ill patient, a cross-table lateral view of the abdomen may demonstrate an aortic aneurysm (see Fig. 1–9). It will not demonstrate dissection or rupture. The availability of emergency ultrasonography may make this examination obsolete.

Pancreatic calcifications may develop with chronic pancreatitis (Fig. 2–14). Occasionally, appendicoliths are seen in the right lower quadrant. These are extremely difficult to differentiate from fecaliths anywhere in the large intestine. The diagnosis of appendicitis should not be based on the presence of a possible appendicolith. If this finding is seen in association with evidence of localized ileus (sentinel loop), the diagnosis of appendicitis is much more likely.

Of course, bone is radiopaque. The vertebral bodies and the lower ribs and upper pelvis can be seen on these radiographs; however, other views are far superior for evaluating these structures. On occasion, a spine fracture is first picked up on a plain abdominal film, in which case further radiologic evaluation is in order.

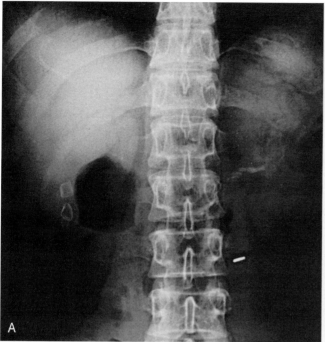

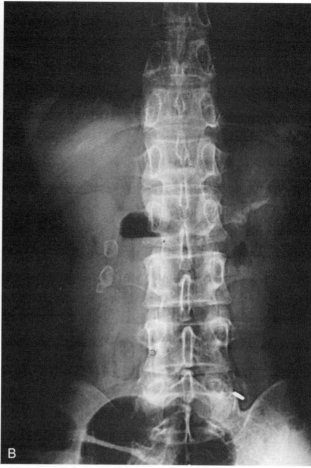

Figure 2–11
Rim-calcified gallstones in the right upper quadrant seen on two frontal views.

Figure 2–12
Gallbladder wall calcification ("porcelain gall-bladder"). Two rim-calcified gallstones are also present.

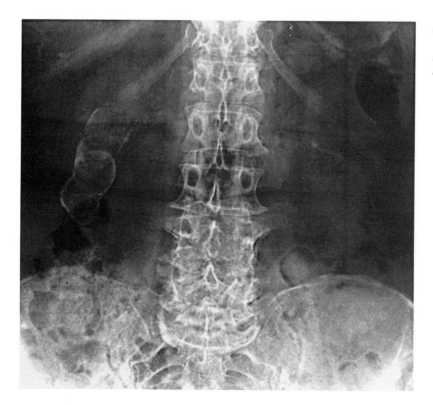

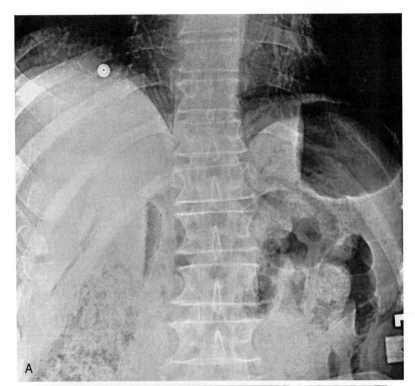

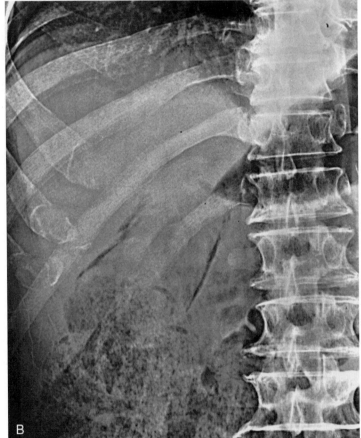

Figure 2–13

Emphysematous cholecystitis, frontal (A) *and decubitus* (B) *views. Note air-fluid level in gallbladder and in gallbladder wall.*

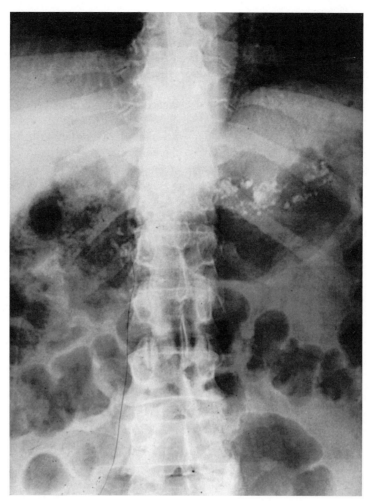

Figure 2-14
Pancreatic calcifications consistent with chronic pancreatitis.

Pneumoperitoneum

Free air in the peritoneum indicates rupture of a hollow viscus. Most of these patients are clinically ill and have evidence of peritonitis on physical examination. Air may be visualized beneath the diaphragm in an upright film (Figs. 2–15, 2–16) or between the abdominal wall and the liver in the left side–down lateral decubitus films. When patients are too ill or cannot be positioned for an upright film, lateral decubitus views should be taken, but an upright chest radiograph is generally recommended for investigation of pneumoperitoneum.

A number of signs of pneumoperitoneum have been described for supine films.[7] They include localized gas in the right upper quadrant, Rigler's sign (gas in intra- and extraluminal spaces outlining the bowel wall), and outlining of the falciform ligament by gas.

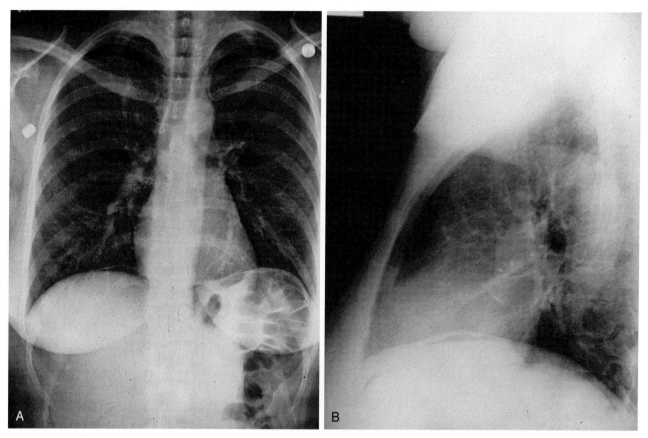

Figure 2-15
Free peritoneal air is seen under the diaphragm on frontal and lateral chest projections. (A) Lucency is seen between the diaphragm and the liver and along the right anteromedial hemidiaphragm. Air is also seen on the lateral projection (B) under the dome of the right hemidiaphragm and anteriorly in the left hemidiaphragm.

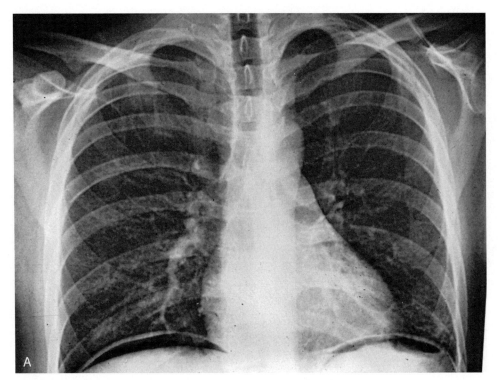

Figure 2–16
Large amount of free intraperitoneal air is seen under the diaphragm on the frontal (A) *and lateral* (B) *chest projections.*

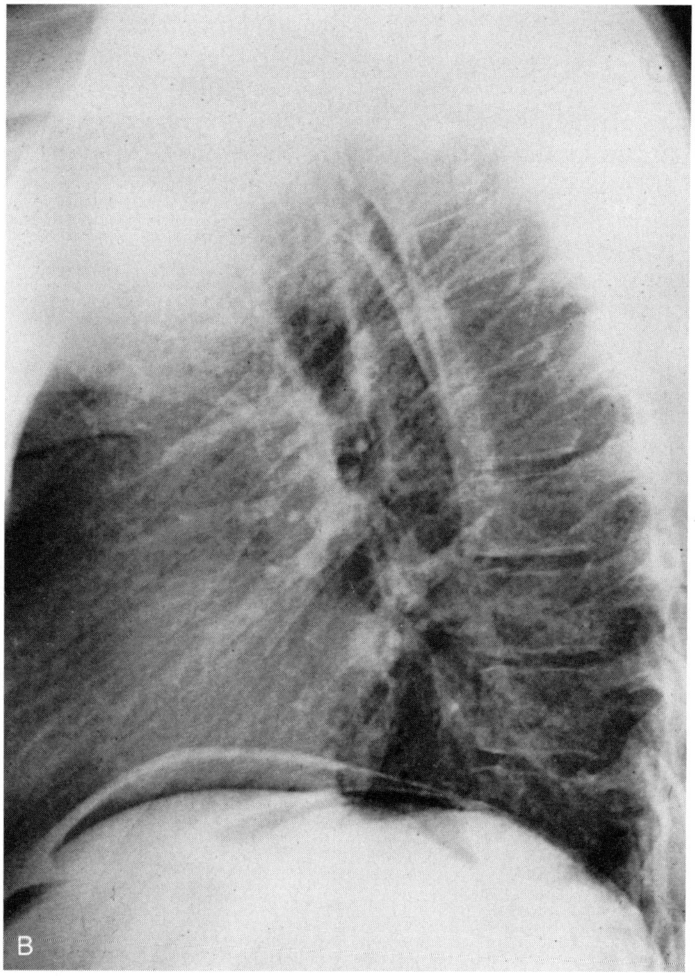

Figure 2–16 (Continued)

Foreign Bodies

Metallic foreign bodies are easily identified. Frontal and lateral views are helpful in localizing them to the esophagus or trachea (Fig. 2–17). The position of an intraabdominal object may be unclear (Fig. 2–18). Nonmetallic objects, such as a toothbrush or a pencil, may also be visible (Figs. 2–19, 2–20). Objects may be followed radiographically as they pass through the gastrointestinal tract (Fig. 2–21).

Text continued on page 82

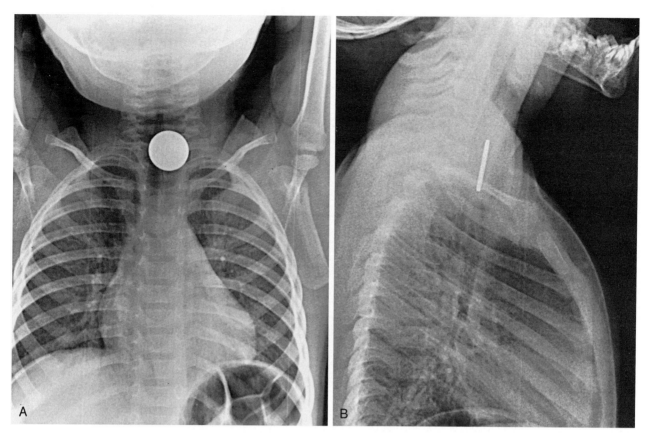

Figure 2–17
A coin is lodged in the esophagus at the lower cervical–upper thoracic level. (A) Frontal view;
(B) lateral view.

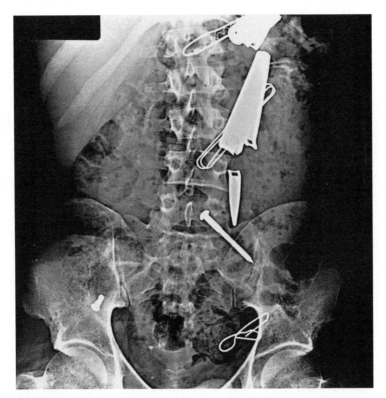

Figure 2–18
Numerous swallowed metallic foreign bodies.

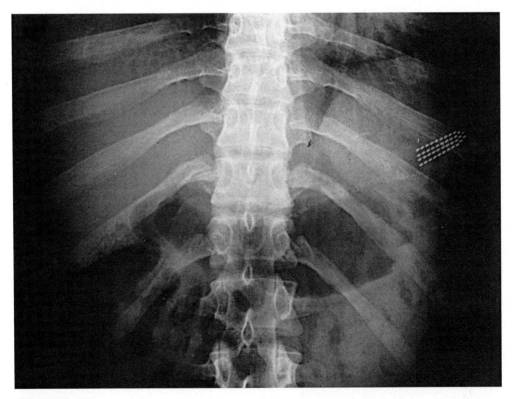

Figure 2–19
Foreign body in the stomach. A toothbrush with radiopaque bristles lies in the gastric fundus. Suture line present just below the foreign body shows that this is a recurring problem.

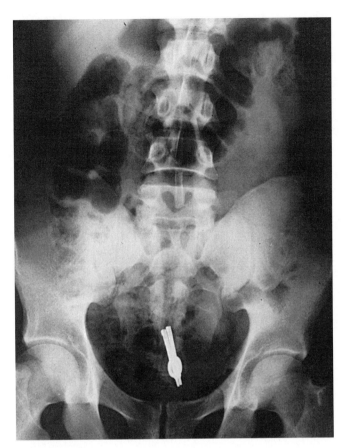

Figure 2–20
Rectal foreign body. Handcuff keys have been secreted in the patient's rectum. Two radiolucent lines next to the keys represent a pencil the patient used to manipulate the keys.

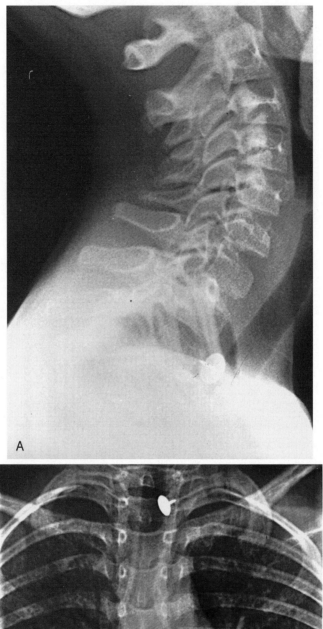

Figure 2–21
Foreign body. A tack is visualized in the upper thoracic esoph-agus (A, B) *and later in the in the abdomen* (C, D).

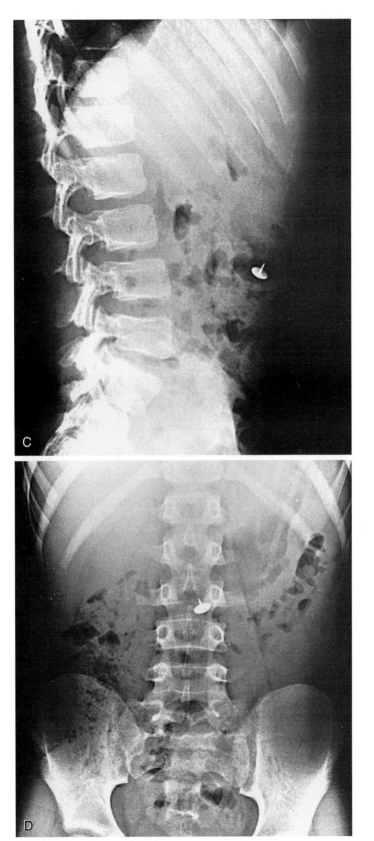

Figure 2–21 (Continued)

Soft Tissues

The solid organs may be seen on plain abdominal radiographs. An enlarged liver or spleen may be seen as a soft tissue density in the appropriate anatomic area, causing mass effect. The borders of the kidneys are often seen on abdominal films; however, extensive hepatomegaly or splenomegaly should be palpable on physical examination. Plain radiographs do not help to identify the cause.

Gallbladder disease often produces no plain film abnormalities. However, gas may be seen in the wall of the gallbladder (as in emphysematous cholecystitis) or in the pericholecystic tissues. Gas may also appear in the biliary tree. Calcification of the gallbladder may give the appearance of a porcelain gallbladder. Calcification is associated with many carcinomas.

In a trauma patient, a pelvic hematoma may be identified by its mass effect. The bowel is pushed up out of the pelvis where it normally lies. Such a hematoma may give an indication of extensive bleeding into the retroperitoneum. Bladder distention also forces the pelvic contents up into the abdomen.

A large soft tissue tumor may likewise give the appearance of mass effect. The edges of the tumor may not be visualized, but abdominal contents are shifted out of their usual positions.

REFERENCES

1. Eisenberg RL, Heineken P, et al: Evaluation of plain abdominal radiographs in the diagnosis of abdominal pain. Ann Surg 1983;197(4):464–469.

2. Campbell JP, Gunn AA: Plain abdominal radiographs and acute abdominal pain. Br J Surg 1988;75(6):554–556.

3. Rothrock SG, Green SM, et al: Plain abdominal radiography in the detection of acute medical and surgical disease in children: A retrospective analysis. Pediatr Emerg Care 1991;7(5):281–285.

4. Mirvis SE, Young JW, et al: Plain film evaluation of patients with abdominal pain: Are three radiographs necessary? AJR 1986;147(3):501–503.

5. Seibert JJ, Parvey LS: The telltale triangle: Use of the supine cross table lateral radiograph of the abdomen in early detection of pneumoperitoneum. Pediatr Radiol 1977;5(4):209–210.

6. Patel NH, Lauber PR: The meaning of a nonspecific abdominal gas pattern. Acad Radiol 1995;2(8):667–669.

7. Levine MS, Scheiner JD, et al: Diagnosis of pneumoperitoneum on supine abdominal radiographs. AJR 1991;156(4):731–735.

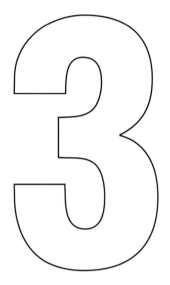

Skull and Facial Radiography

GARY A. JOHNSON, MD

Skull

Since a large percentage of emergency department patients present with head trauma of varying degrees, skull radiographs can frequently be ordered. The vast majority of these patients, however, can be managed without plain skull radiography.

Masters and colleagues[1] have developed a management strategy for patients whose clinical presentation indicates low risk for intracerebral complications. The low-risk group included patients who had complaints of headaches, dizziness, scalp hematoma, scalp laceration or abrasion, and no depressed level of consciousness, focal neurologic signs, or penetrating skull injury. Patients with neurologic signs (the high-risk group) were candidates for both emergency computed tomography (CT) and neurosurgery consultation. Plain skull radiography was not helpful for this group. Patients with a penetrating skull injury or depressed fracture tend to have a history that makes these lesions obvious (e.g., gunshot wound, blow with a pointed object like a hammer or a rod; Fig. 3–1). Skull films may help the neurosurgeon in surgical repair of depressed fractures found by physical exam or CT; however, most patients can be appropriately managed without plain skull radiographs.

Indications for pediatric skull radiography are largely untested in the literature. Infants are more difficult to assess neurologically, and, therefore, many practitioners have a lower threshold for obtaining skull films for infants with suspected head injuries.

Interpretation of skull radiographs can be difficult because of multiple markings in a normal skull, including suture lines and vascular markings. Distinguishing fractures from normal markings can be based on the shape of the path (fractures tend to be much straighter than either vascular markings or sutures) and by location (Figs. 3–2, 3–3). Both vascular markings and sutures tend to have predictable distributions. Interpretation can be made more complicated by the fact that fractures may occur through sutures (diastatic fractures).

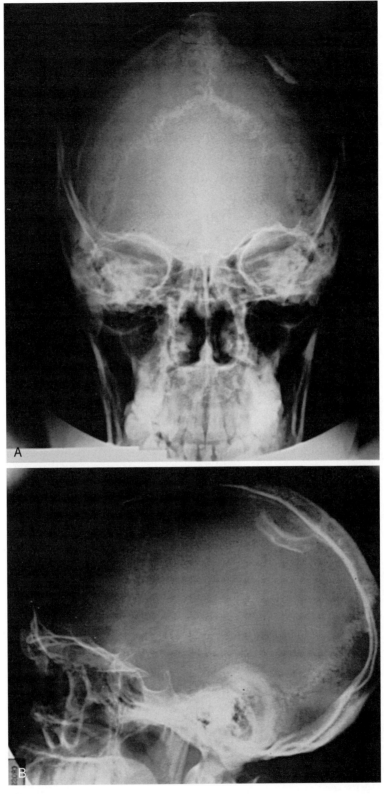

Figure 3–1
Depressed skull fracture seen on (A) frontal and (B) lateral projections. This patient was hit with a ball-peen hammer, and an indentation with the shape of the ball is visible.

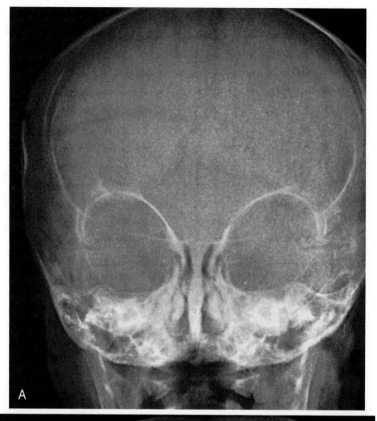

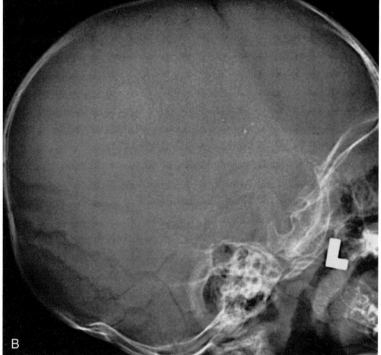

Figure 3–2
Linear fracture of the posterior aspect of the parietal bone seen on (A) frontal and (B) lateral views. The fracture is relatively straight, whereas the lambdoid sutures have a much more serpiginous course with the typical interdigitating appearance.

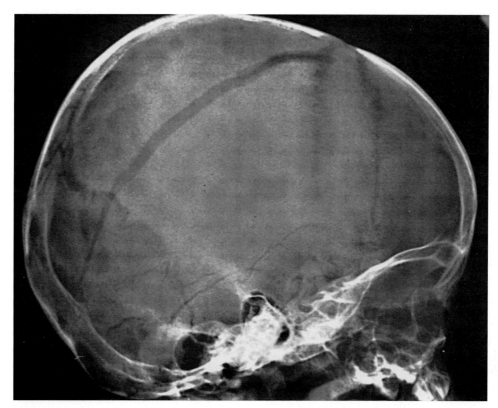

Figure 3–3
Parietal bone fracture.

Maxillofacial Radiography

Maxillofacial radiography can be considered for patients with facial trauma or possible paranasal sinus disease (Fig. 3–4). An adequate maxillofacial x-ray series includes Caldwell, Waters, and lateral views. Other views may be considered in certain clinical situations. These views include orbital oblique films, zygomatic arch films, and nasal bone films. The mandible can be examined with either a series of plain films or a single panoramic view.

Different views can highlight various regions of the face. On a Caldwell view the petrous bone overlaps the inferior aspect of the orbits, and the frontal and ethmoid sinuses are seen well. On Waters' view the petrous bone is shifted downward, which allows visualization of inferior and medial orbital floors and the maxillary and ethmoid sinuses. The lateral radiograph also allows visualization of the ethmoid, sphenoid, and maxillary sinuses and provides an excellent view of the anterior and posterior walls of the frontal sinus. A separate technique is required to adequately visualize the nasal bone.

Reading maxillofacial films for trauma involves tracing cortical bone lines of the orbit, zygomatic arch, nasal bone, maxilla, and mandible. An effusion in a paranasal sinus can be an indication of a fracture (Fig. 3–5). Knowledge of common fracture patterns can greatly enhance interpretation. Blowout fractures of the orbit tend to involve a fracture of the inferior or medial orbital wall. These are often caused by a blow to the globe that transmits this force to the orbital wall and produces a fracture. An inferior blowout fracture can be manifested as a "hanging drop" of soft tissue protruding into the maxillary sinus. Zygomaticomaxillary fractures are commonly called "tripod fractures" (Fig. 3–6). These fractures occur at the zygomatic arch, the lateral orbit (zygomaticofrontal suture), and the zygomaticomaxillary suture.

Nasal bone and mandibular fractures may require specialized views. Mandibular views may be performed with routine plain radiography (Fig. 3–7) or a panoramic view. Nasal bones are best seen with lateral coned-down views (Fig. 3–8).

LeFort fractures have been described as three separate fracture lines (Fig. 3–9). LeFort I is a fracture along the maxilla at the nasal floor. This allows the entire maxillary dental ridge to move independently of the rest of the face. LeFort II is a fracture through the maxilla, up through the orbit and nasal bones, and down to the contralateral maxilla. This allows the nose and upper teeth to move as a unit independent of the rest of the face (pyramidal disassociation). LeFort III (craniofacial disassociation) is a fracture through the zygomatic arch, orbits, and nasal bones bilaterally. This allows the entire face to move independently of the skull. It is important to note that patients often present with a partial LeFort fracture and do not always show all manifestations of the classic fracture.

What constitutes the appropriate clinical and radiologic approach to facial trauma is unclear. Manson and coworkers[2] studied CT scans to identify precise fracture patterns. They found CT useful for early detection of facial fracture in high-energy injuries. They found that CT examination of these trauma patients enabled physicians to coordinate operating schedules and prioritize injuries. They also found that when fractures could not be assessed by physical examination (e.g., medial orbit or posterior wall of frontal sinus), CT produced benefits.

Finkel[3] looked at physical examination, CT, and plain radiography and found CT to be superior. No information on clinical significance of the fractures was given. Thai and colleagues[4] found that physical examination can reliably assess the facial bones; however, CT was beneficial in the management of orbital fractures. Gautam and Leonard[5] found that patients with a head injury, even a minor injury, very often had coexisting facial bone fractures. They recommend that facial fractures be sought "clinically and radiologically" when a minor head injury is discovered.

Pediatric craniofacial fractures are somewhat different. Koltai and associates[6] found that children younger than 7 years had a higher incidence of superior orbit fractures as compared with the usual adult fracture patterns of medial or inferior orbit injury.

Soft tissue neck films are useful for detecting foreign bodies (Fig. 3–10), retropharyngeal lesions (Fig. 3–11), and epiglottitis (Fig. 3–12).

Text continued on page 100

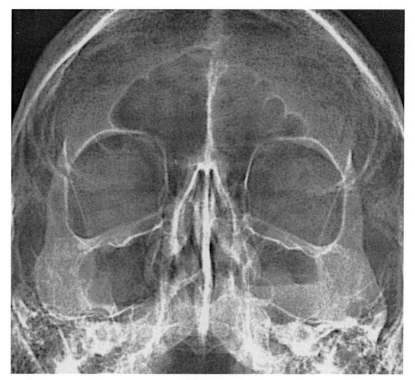

Figure 3–4

Acute sinusitis. Upright Waters' view shows air-fluid level in the left maxillary sinus.

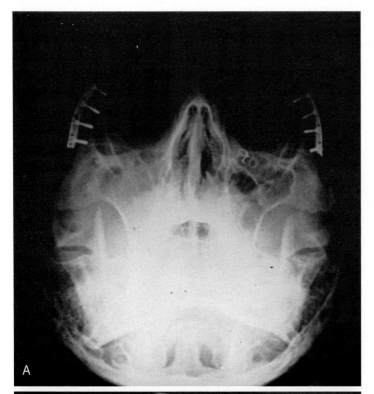

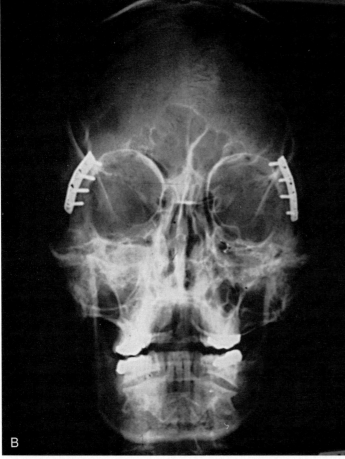

Figure 3–5
Right orbital floor and medial orbit fracture. Opacification of the right maxillary sinus is seen on Waters' view (A). (B) Frontal (Caldwell's) view shows right orbital emphysema. Bilateral metal plates and left orbital floor wire show that trauma is often a recurrent disease.

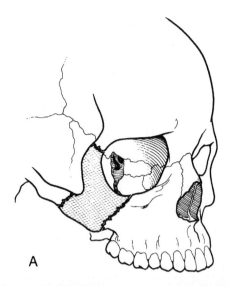

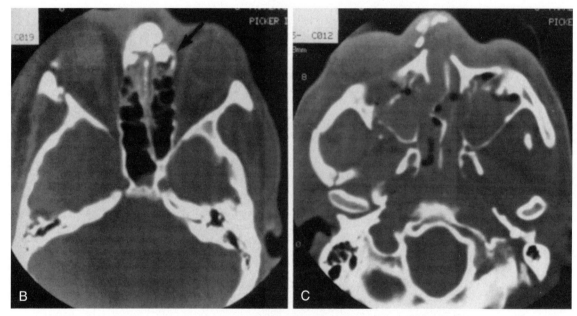

Figure 3–6

(A) *A diagram showing a tripod fracture. The stippled area indicates the segment of bone that has been separated from the facial strut. Note the zygomatic, the inferior orbital, and the lateral orbital components of the fracture.* (B) *This transaxial image shows the lateral orbital component of a tripod fracture in a patient who suffered a complex facial injury. Notice also the fracture of the nasoethmoid complex* (arrow). (C) *An image taken slightly lower shows a compound fracture of the zygoma. Note again the nasoethmoid complex fracture. (Redman HC, Ruddy PD, Miller GL, Rollins NK: Emergency Radiology. Philadelphia: WB Saunders, 1993.)*

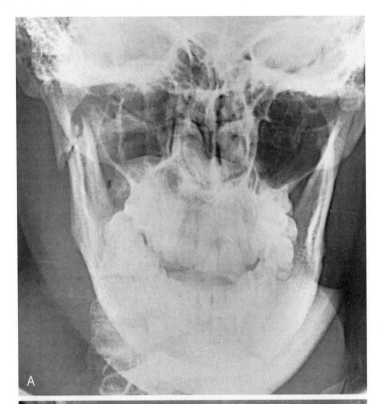

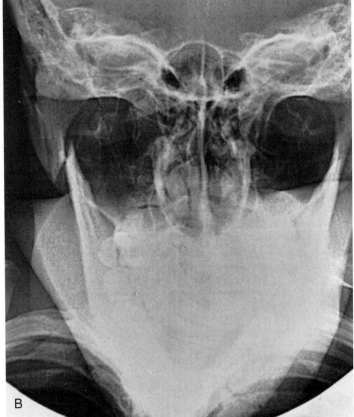

Figure 3–7
Mandibular condyle fracture with a parasymphyseal fracture on the contralateral side is seen on frontal (A, B) and lateral (C) views.

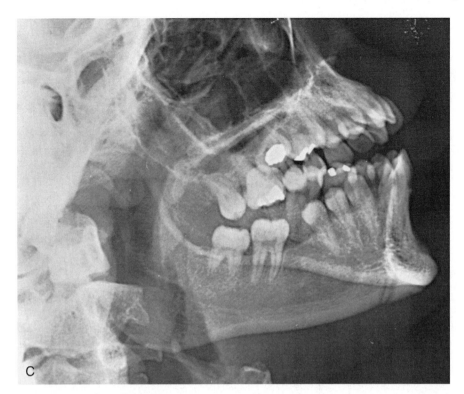

Figure 3–7 (Continued)

Figure 3–8
Nasal bone and anterior nasal spine fractures.

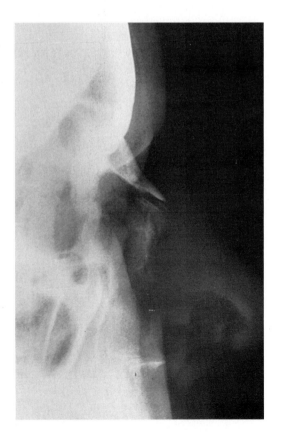

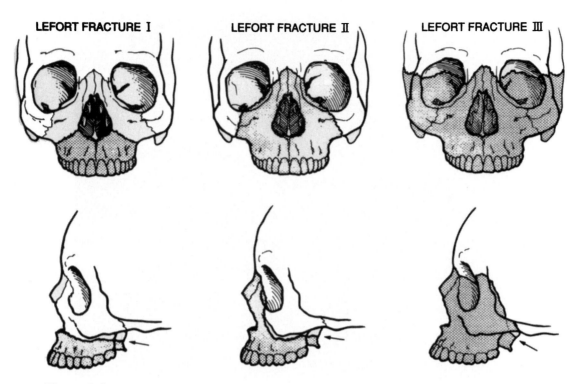

LEFORT FRACTURE I   **LEFORT FRACTURE II**   **LEFORT FRACTURE III**

Figure 3–9
This class of midface fractures has three subcategories, which are numbered I, II, and III. In the LeFort I fracture, the alveolar ridge is separated from the maxilla, but the nasal and orbital areas are not involved. In the LeFort II fracture, there is involvement of the medial orbital areas and the nasal bone, but the fracture does not extend through the lateral orbits and the zygoma. In the LeFort III fracture, also known as a midface separation, the fracture extends through the medial and lateral orbital walls and the zygoma, and the midface is essentially freed from the skull in terms of its bony attachments. In this illustration these fractures are shown as stippled areas. Note the extension of the fracture through the pterygoid plate in all three types (arrows). (Redman HC, Purdy PD, Miller GL, Rollins NK: Emergency Radiology. Philadelphia: WB Saunders, 1993.)

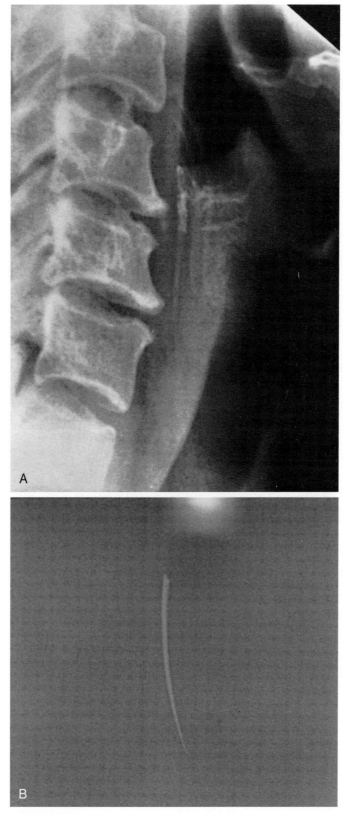

Figure 3–10
Chicken bone in cervical esophagus. (A) Vertical linear density anterior to cervical vertebral bodies. (B) Photograph of the bone following removal.

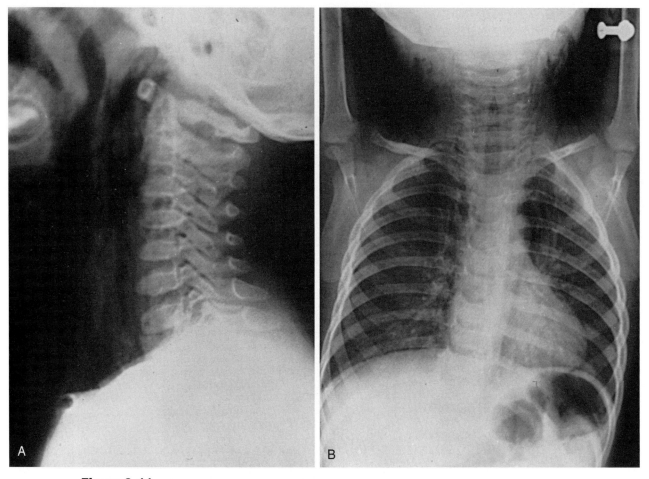

Figure 3–11
Retropharyngeal abscess. Air in the retropharyngeal and mediastinal tissues is seen on lateral neck (A) and chest (B) radiographs. This is the result of a puncture wound to the posterior pharynx.

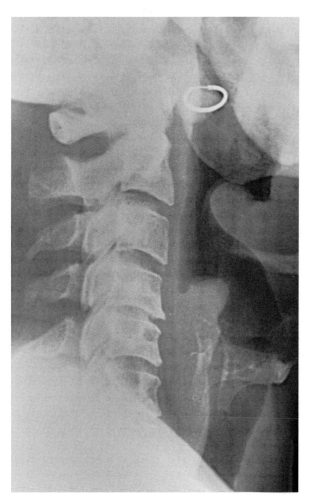

Figure 3–12
Epiglottitis. Neck film of the soft tissues reveals marked thickening of the epiglottis.

REFERENCES

1. Masters SJ, et al: Skull x-ray examinations after head trauma. N Engl J Med 1987;316(2):84–91.

2. Manson PN, et al: Toward CT-based facial fracture treatment. Plast Reconstr Surg 1990;85:202.

3. Finkel DR, Ringler SL, et al: Comparison of the diagnostic methods used in maxillofacial trauma. Plast Reconstr Surg 1985;75:32.

4. Thai KN, Hummel RP, et al: The role of computed tomographic scanning in the management of facial trauma. J Trauma 1997;43(2):214–218.

5. Gautam V, Leonard EA: Bony injuries in association with minor head injury: Lessons for improving the diagnosis of facial fractures. Injury 1994;25(1):47–49.

6. Koltai PJ, Amjad I, et al: Orbital fractures in children. Arch Otolaryngol 1995;121(12):1375–1379.

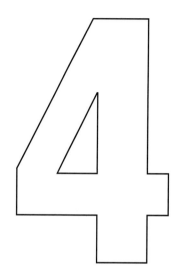

Spine
Radiography

GARY A. JOHNSON, MD

CERVICAL SPINE

The cervical spine should be considered to include the cranium, all seven cervical vertebrae, and the first thoracic vertebra. The vertebral bodies and cartilaginous discs generally bear compressive load. Ligaments and posterior bony elements lend stability on stretching. Three vertical columns are considered in assessing the stability of the spine. The anterior column consists of the anterior two thirds of the vertebral body; the middle column extends from the posterior third of the vertebral body to the spinal laminar line; and the posterior column, from the spinal laminar line to the tip of the spinous process. Unstable injuries generally involve the middle column and one other column.

Mechanism of injury has often been used to understand spine trauma. Extension injuries, flexion injuries, rotational injuries, axial load compression injuries, and lateral flexion injuries have all been described. Flexion injuries may result in ligament disruption and subluxation, compression fractures, flexion teardrop fractures, and bilateral facet dislocations. Extension injuries may cause extension dislocation from ligament rupture, anterior or posterior fractures of the atlas, extension teardrop fractures, or traumatic spondylolisthesis. Compression mechanisms may cause bursting of any vertebral body, including C1 (Jefferson fracture). Lateral flexion may fracture a transverse process or the lateral mass of C1. A classification of fractures based on mechanism is inherently limited by the fact that many fractures have multiple mechanisms, and, often, the description of the mechanism by the patient or first-response caregivers is vague.

What films are appropriate for investigating cervical spine trauma is a matter of debate. Clearly, the patient's overall condition needs to be considered as it relates to procedures of different duration, cost, and inconvenience. Many authors advocate a five-film series with lateral (Fig. 4–1A), AP, odontoid, and oblique projections.[1, 2] Others believe that a three-film series—lateral, AP, and odontoid—(Fig.

4–1B) may be adequate for initial screening.[3, 4] More recent reports[5] have noted that a lateral plain film combined with CT may be the most complete and time-efficient way to assess a multiple trauma victim's cervical spine.

Considerable controversy surrounds the question of the appropriate cervical spine evaluation for patients who are alert and stable and whose symptoms are minimal. Stiell and coworkers[6] noted wide variations in emergency department use of cervical spine radiography. All practitioners diagnosed all cervical spine fractures in their study of 6855 patients. Other authors[7, 8] have found that clinical examination alone cannot reliably assess the cervical spine and detect all fractures after blunt trauma.

The lateral radiograph is the most sensitive for cervical spine injuries. The spine must be examined from the cranium to the cervicothoracic junction. A lateral cervical spine film must be inspected for adequate viewing of the entire spine and for inappropriate rotation. Proper patient positioning will produce a lateral view that superimposes the articular masses of each vertebra. If a lateral mass is seen individually (not superimposed), the film must be rotated or a rotational dislocation must be present.

Often, all the vertebrae from C1 to the cervicothoracic junction cannot be seen on the initial film. Traction applied to both arms may enhance visualization, provided the patient has no painful shoulder or upper extremity injury. Other methods for seeing the C7 and T1 include oblique views and a view with the patient's arm raised (swimmer's view). The patient should not be removed from supine cervical spine immobilization until the clinical and/or radiographic findings have been conclusively determined to be negative.

A pillar view is an oblique view that reveals the articular masses en face and has been advocated for cervical spine visualization.[9] Because the pillar view requires rotating the patient's head, it cannot be used until unstable spine fracture or dislocation has been excluded.

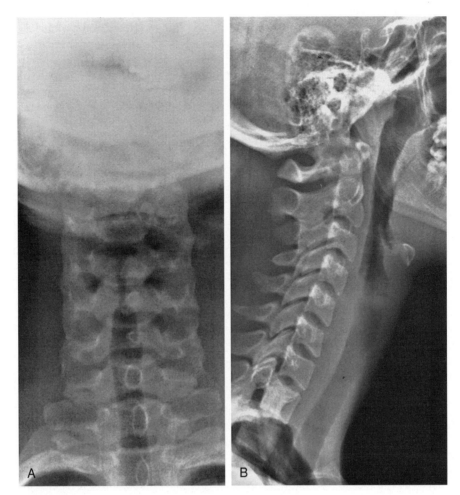

Figure 4–1
Normal (A) AP and (B) lateral cervical spine films.

A mnemonic for interpretation of the lateral cervical spine is *ABCs*: *A* for alignment, *B* for bones, *C* for cartiliage, and *s* for soft tissue space. Alignment can be assessed by four lines: anterior vertebral body, posterior vertebral body, spinal laminar line, and tip of the spinous process line. In addition, Swischuk's lines and atlantooccipital stability must be assessed. Swischuk's line (Fig. 4–2) is the spinal laminar line for the first three vertebrae. The C1-C2 complex allows a great range of motion (Figs. 4–3, 4–4); however, the line should remain constant in all degrees of flexion and extension. In adults, the posterior vertebral body line and spinal laminar line should describe a canal size of approximately 30 mm at C1 and 22 mm from C3 through T1. Bone integrity must be assessed for each verte-bra. The cartilaginous spaces of the intervertebral discs and the predental space must be assessed. The predental space should be constant with flexion and extension of the neck and should be 5 mm or less in children and 3 mm or less in adults (Fig. 4–5).

Inspection of the soft tissue shadow may detect hematoma. Many models for measuring a soft tissue space have been proposed, but no single set of measurements is reliably sensitive and specific. A nasogastric or endotracheal tube may make it difficult to visualize the anterior aspect of the soft tissue shadow, which can make interpretation difficult. Interpretation of the soft tissue shadow should be based much more on contour than on measurements.

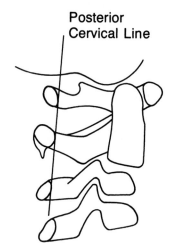

Posterior Cervical Line

Figure 4–2

The posterior cervical line is envisioned as connecting the posterior laminar line of the atlas to the posterior laminar line of C3 and helps to differentiate pseudosubluxation from true subluxation. The posterior laminar line of the axis should normally lie within 1 mm anterior or posterior to the posterior cervical line. (Ellis GL: Imaging of the atlas (C1) and axis (C2). Emerg Med Clin North Am 1991;9:719.)

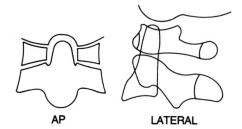

AP　　**LATERAL**

Figure 4–3

The articular relationships of the occiput, atlas, and axis. Because the articular surfaces of the atlas and axis are convex in relation to each other, a great deal of rotation, as well as flexion and extension, is allowed. (Ellis GL: Imaging of the atlas (C1) and axis (C2). Emerg Med Clin North Am 1991;9:719.)

Figure 4–4

The ligamentous relationships unique to the occipitoatlantoaxial region. (Ellis GL: Imaging of the atlas (C1) and axis (C2). Emerg Med Clin North Am 1991;9:719.)

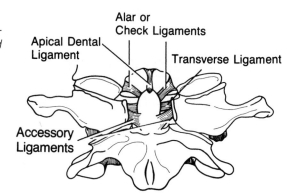

Apical Dental Ligament

Alar or Check Ligaments

Transverse Ligament

Accessory Ligaments

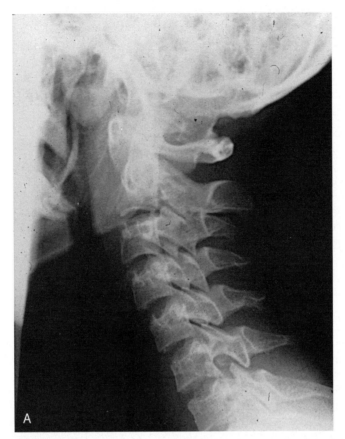

Figure 4–5
Transverse ligament rupture. (A) Lateral film reveals an abnormally wide space between the anterior arch of C1 and the odontoid process of C2. There is soft tissue swelling anterior to the upper cervical spine.

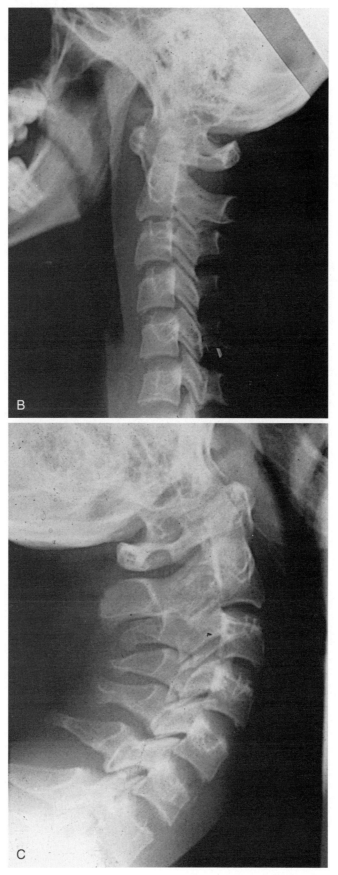

Figure 4–5 Continued
(B) Flexion and (C) extension views show mobility of C1 on C2.

SPECIFIC INJURIES

Atlantooccipital dislocation is a dislocation of the skull relative to the cervical vertebrae (Fig. 4–6). The C1-C2 complex will not be articulated normally at the foramen magnum.

Jefferson's fracture is a burst fracture of C1 that commonly results from an axial force down the cervical spine. This fracture may be difficult to identify on a single lateral radiograph and is often best seen on an open-mouth odontoid view. Such a view shows fracture and displacement of the lateral masses of C1 (Figs. 4–7, 4–8). Lower cervical fractures may be associated with Jefferson's fracture.

Odontoid fractures are relatively common. The dens of the odontoid bone provides much rotational range of motion, but it is vulnerable to fracture (Fig. 4–9), often with hyperflexion. Odontoid fractures have been divided into three subtypes. Type I is an avulsion of the tip of the dens (odontoid process). Type II is a fracture through the junction of the dens and C2. A type III fracture extends through the vertebral body. Like Jefferson's fractures, odontoid fractures may be difficult to see on a single lateral film, and the odontoid view or CT is often necessary to fully evaluate the odontoid process and the body of C2 (Figs. 4–10 through 4–13).

Hangman's fracture is a fracture of a portion of both articular masses at C2 and is most accurately considered "traumatic spondylolisthesis" (Figs. 4–14, 4–15). It most often involves the pars interarticularis and often results from hyperflexion, as with rapid deceleration in a motor vehicle accident. This fracture is unstable, but neurologic injury is often avoided owing to the fact that the spinal canal is relatively wide at the level of C2.

Compression fractures (burst fractures) (Figs. 4–16 through 4–20) often result from axial loading or hyperflexion. A lateral film may show a fracture line, loss of vertical height of the vertebral body, or bone fragments. Compression fractures are at times difficult to distinguish from burst injuries. Posterior dislocation of bone or soft tissue fragments commonly causes neurologic injuries (see Fig. 4–20 and 4–21).

Teardrop fractures (Fig. 4–22) and dislocations commonly are caused by axial compression and either flexion or extension. Avulsion of the anteroinferior aspect of the vertebral body may appear relatively unremarkable; however, the anterior and posterior ligaments typically are disrupted and thus the fracture is unstable. Neurologic injury is common.

Facet dislocations can be unilateral or bilateral. Bilateral dislocations are generally well visualized on a single lateral film (Fig. 4–23). Anterior dislocation of the superior aspect of the spine is evident, and the superior facet is generally easily seen to be anterior to the inferior facet joint. Unilateral facet dislocation may be difficult to see on the initial plain film. There is generally less than 25% anterior subluxation of the superior vertebral body. A frontal plain film may show rotational asymmetry of the spinous processes. Oblique views may be very helpful in showing the dislocation and the facet fracture.

Spinous process fractures are common. A C7 spinous process fracture is usually called "clay shoveler's fracture" (Fig. 4–24). These injuries are generally stable when they occur in isolation. Os odontoideum is a normal variant that can be mistaken for a fracture (Fig. 4–25).

Text continued on page 128

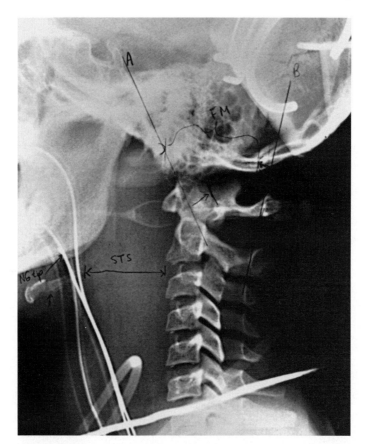

Figure 4–6

Anterior occipitoatlantal dislocation. The skull is shifted forward in relation to the spine. There is widening of the distance between the occipital condyles and the lateral masses of C1. In normal cervical spine the clivus-to-foramen magnum line intersects the tip of the odontoid process (line A). The spinolaminal line (line B) should intersect the posterior aspect of the foramen magnum (FM). Soft tissue swelling (STS) is marked. NG tip, nasogastric tube.

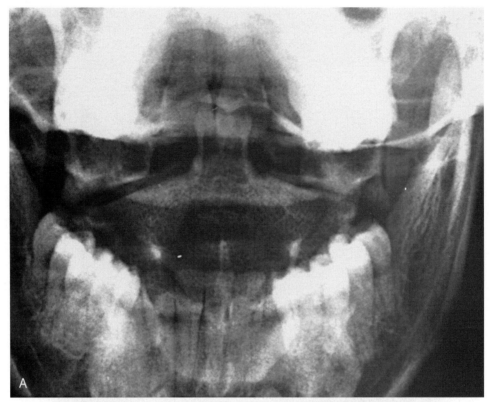

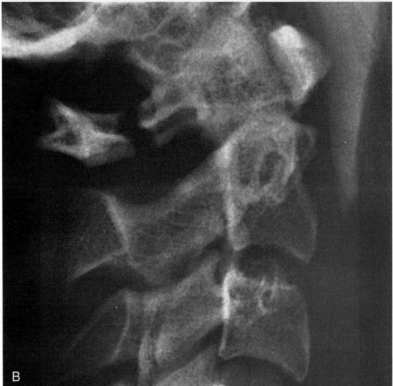

Figure 4-7
Jefferson's fracture. (A) Open-mouth view shows unusually wide distance between the lateral masses of C1 with respect to the dens and lateral displacement with respect to the lateral masses of C2. (B) Lateral view shows a fracture of the posterior arch of C1.

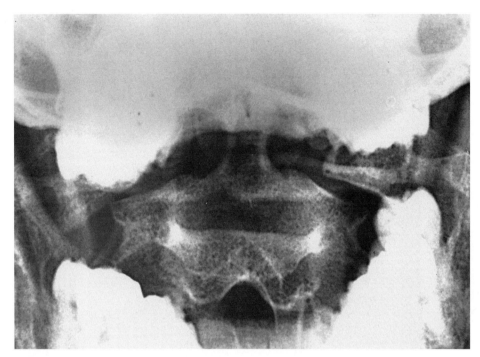

Figure 4–8
Jefferson's fracture. AP radiograph reveals lateral displacement of both C1 lateral masses.

Figure 4–9
Anderson-D'Alonzo classification of dens fractures. (Ellis GL: Imaging of the atlas (C1) and axis (C2). Emerg Med Clin North Am 1991;9:719.)

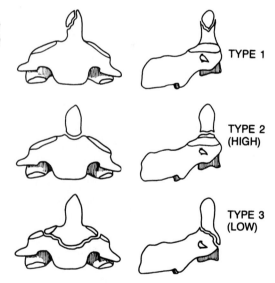

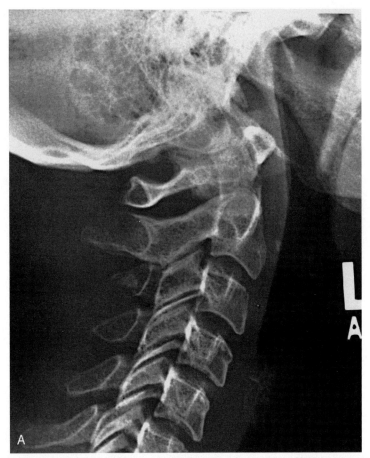

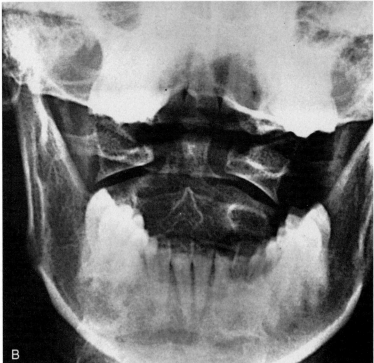

Figure 4–10

Odontoid fracture. Type II odontoid fracture at the base of the dens. (A) The lateral view reveals anterior cortical interruption with very slight posterior angulation of the dens. (B) Open-mouth view shows fracture line at base of dens.

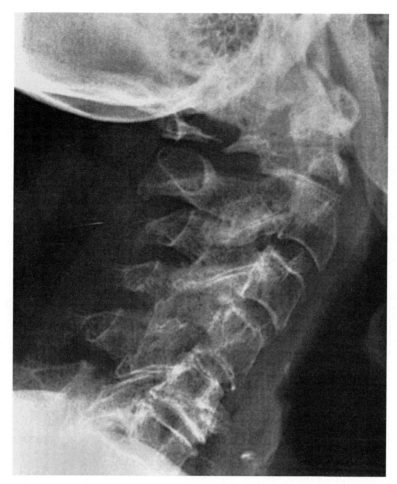

Figure 4–11
Type III odontoid fracture involves the body of C2 with posterior angulation of the dens. Fracture of the posterior arch of C1 is also evident.

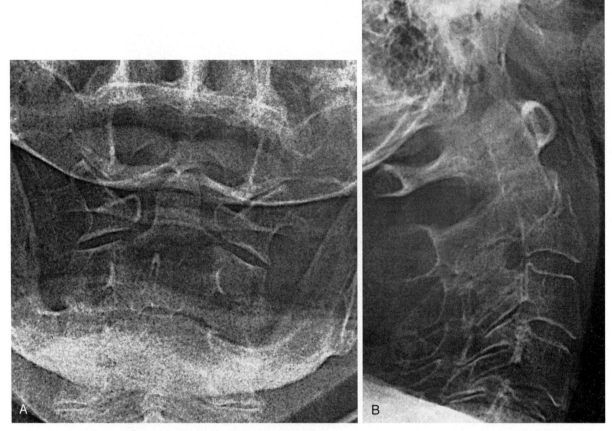

Figure 4–12
Type III odontoid fracture with posterior displacement of dens seen on (A) *open month and* (B) *lateral views.*

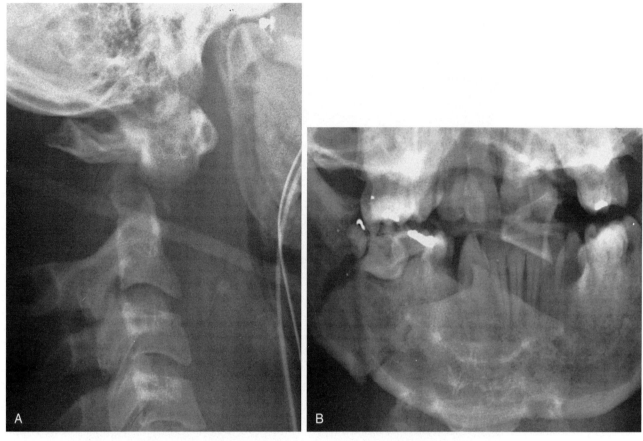

Figure 4–13
Atlantoaxial fracture dislocation. (A) Lateral and (B) open-mouth views demonstrate fractures of the dens and right lateral mass of C1 with marked atlantoaxial distraction and anterior dislocation. A right mandibular fracture is also identified.

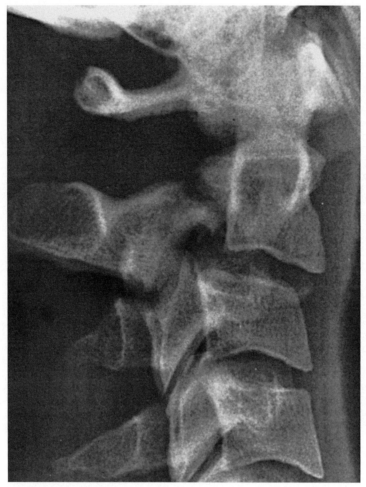

Figure 4–14

Hangman's fracture. There is a pars interarticularis fracture with anterior subluxation of C2 on C3.

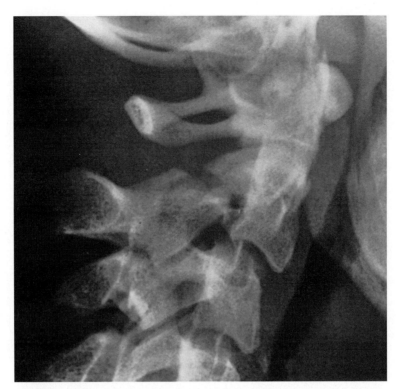

Figure 4–15
Hangman's fracture. Pars interarticularis fracture of C2 with anterior displacement of C1 and the body of C2 in relation to C3.

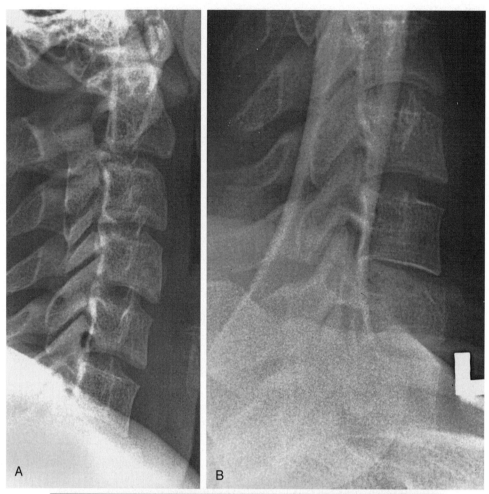

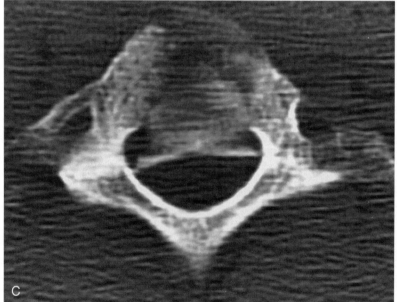

Figure 4–16

(A) *Initial lateral film shows C1–C6 vertebral bodies only.* (B) *Swimmer's view shows compression fracture of C7 but no evidence of retropulsion.* (C) *CT shows retropulsed fracture fragment.*

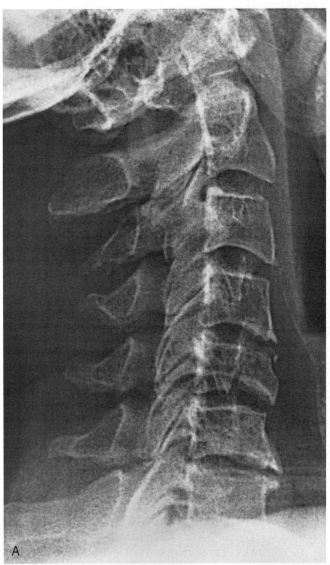

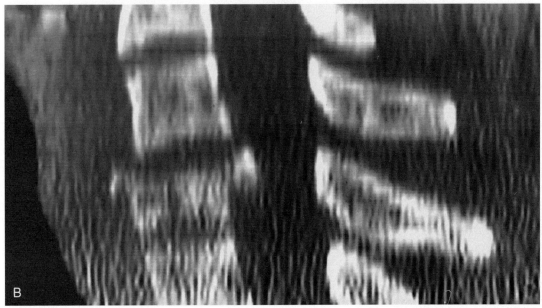

Figure 4–17
Burst fracture of C5 with retropulsion of small fragment. (A) Lateral plain film and (B) sagittal reconstruction CT images.

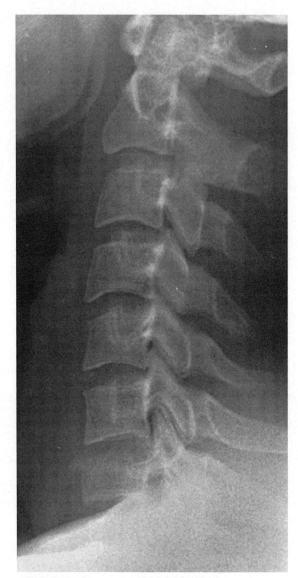

Figure 4–18
C7 compression fracture. The height of the C7 verte-bral body is less than that of C6.

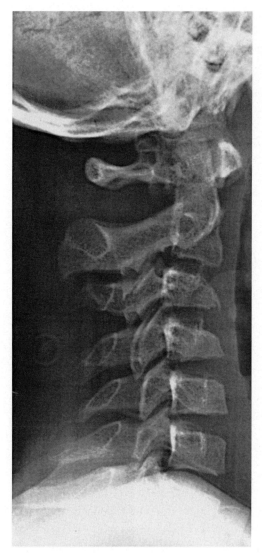

Figure 4–19
Mild compression fracture of C3 and C4.

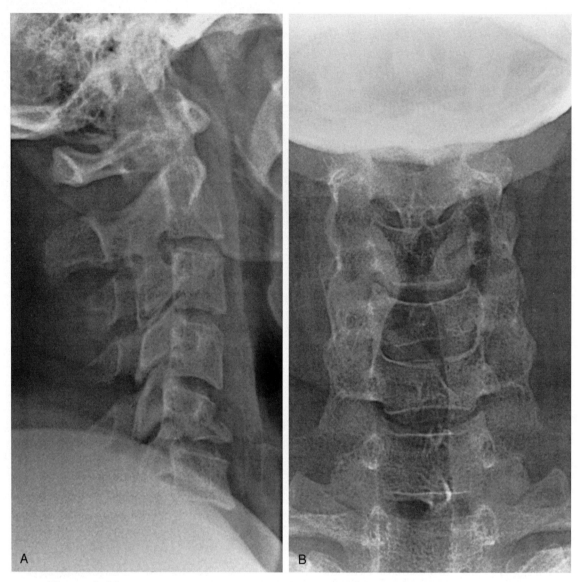

Figure 4–20
Compression fracture of C5. (A) Some posterior subluxation of C5, as compared to C6, is seen on the lateral view. (B) There is widening of the distance between interspinous processes C4 and C5. This is compatible with the posterior ligament injury.

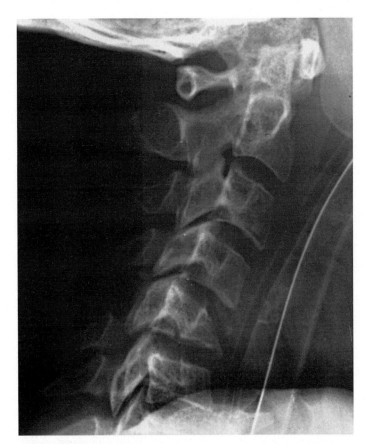

Figure 4–21
C5 vertebral body fracture with posterior subluxation, kyphosis, and an inferiorly displaced laminar fracture.

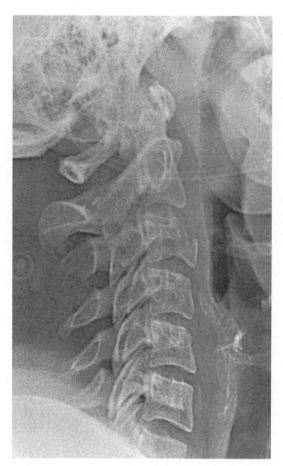

Figure 4–22
Extension teardrop fracture of C3.

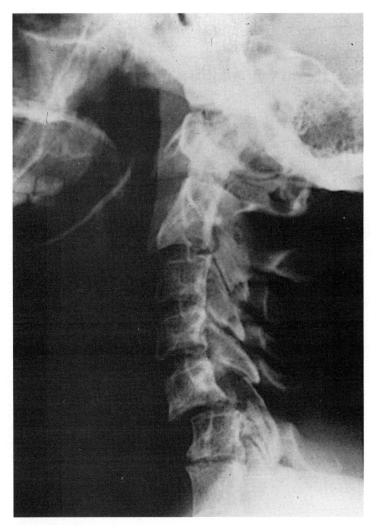

Figure 4-23
Subluxation of C5 on C6 secondary to a ligament injury. The C5 inferior facets are perched on the superior facets of the body of C6. There is no evidence of bone injury.

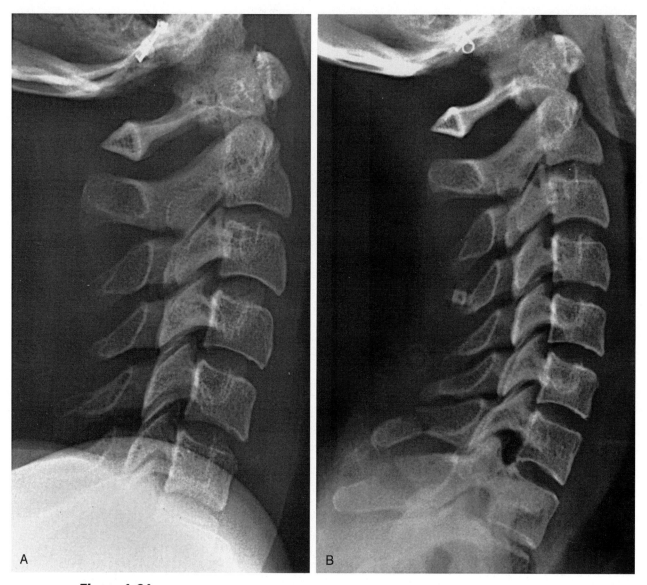

Figure 4–24

C7 and T1 spinous process fracture. (A) Initial lateral view extends to the top of the C7 vertebral body. (B) Repeat lateral view that includes the top of T2 demonstrates C2 and T1 spinous process fracture. These lesions have been called "clay shoveler's fractures."

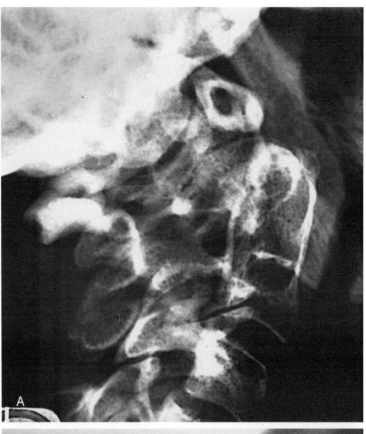

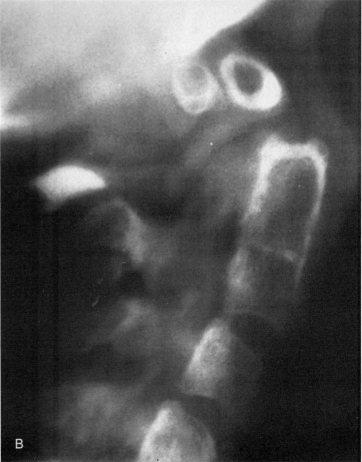

Figure 4–25
Os odontoideum. Smooth, well-corticated bone ossicle superior to C2 and posterior to the anterior arch of C1 seen on (A) plain film and (B) tomogram.

THORACOLUMBAR SPINE

The thoracic spine is splinted by the rib cage but still can absorb enough force to fracture. The upper thoracic spine (T1–T10) benefits most from the rib cage, but twisting or shearing forces can cause fractures or dislocations. As in the cervical spine, axial compression can cause compression fractures, but burst fractures are much less common. A powerful perpendicular force (often from behind) may cause disruption of the posterior ligaments, and sometimes fracture of the facet joints. If the column remains out of alignment, traumatic spondylolisthesis results. These injuries are often associated with neurologic injury, since the thoracic spinal canal is relatively narrow.

The thoracolumbar junction (T11–L2) is most vulnerable to hyperflexion injuries. This area has the greatest range of motion of the entire thoracolumbar spine. A vertebral compression fracture (Fig. 4–26) is not uncommon after an axial load. A great axial load may cause a vertebral burst fracture (Fig. 4–27) with involvement of both anterior and middle columns. Flexion or lateral bending can also fracture the transverse processes (Fig. 4–28).

The thoracolumbar area is susceptible to seatbelt injuries. A powerful force may throw the patient's body forward, and a deceleration injury may be concentrated at the level of the lumbar spine. A fracture that extends horizontally through the vertebral body and posterior elements is commonly referred to as "Chance's fracture" (Fig. 4–29). Posterior ligamentous disruption is common with this injury, as are neurologic injuries.

Many trauma centers routinely obtain thoracolumbar spine radiographs of patients who have significant blunt force trauma. Samuels and Kerstein[10] reviewed blunt trauma cases and asserted that the physical examination could reliably rule out injury in asymptomatic, alert patients. Meldon and Moettus,[11] who reviewed 145 patients with thoracolumbar fractures, drew the same conclusion.

Inflammatory changes may be seen in the lumbar spine. Ankylosing spondylitis (Fig. 4–30) may present as "bamboo spine" with syndesmophyte formation.

Text continued on page 134

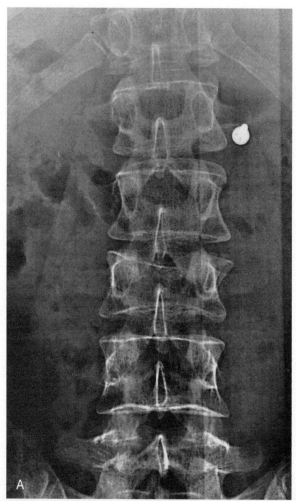

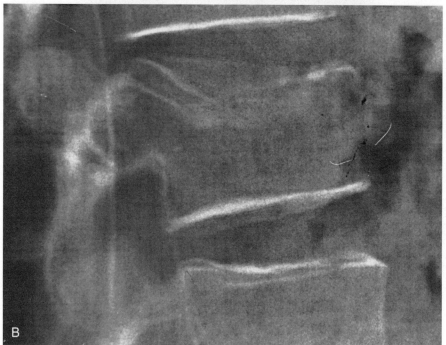

Figure 4–26
L3 compression fracture, (A) frontal and (B) lateral views.

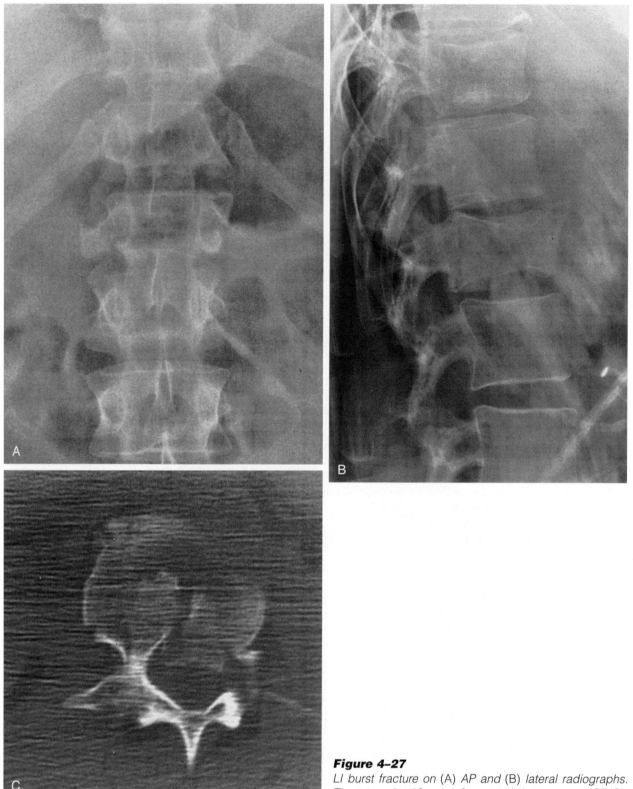

Figure 4–27
*LI burst fracture on (A) AP and (B) lateral radiographs.
The retropulsed fracture fragment is best seen on CT (C).*

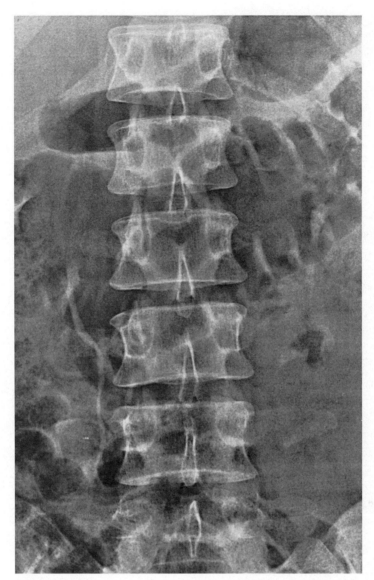

Figure 4–28
Left transverse process fractures.

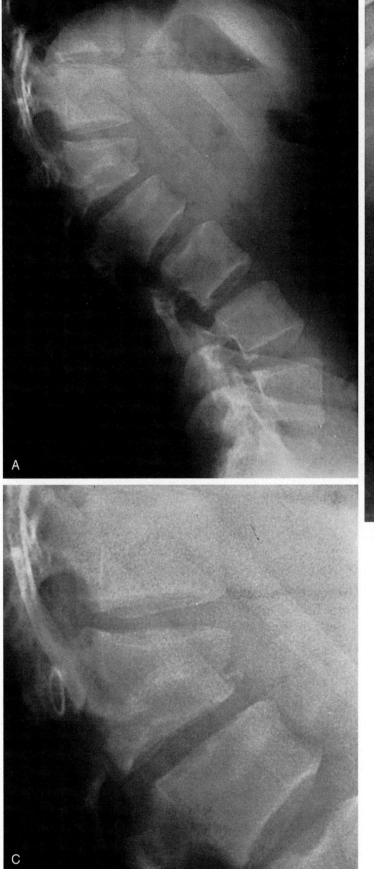

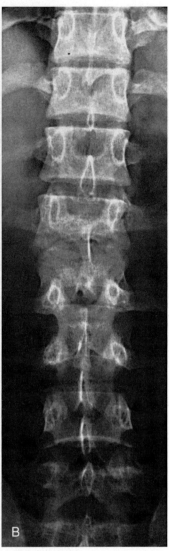

Figure 4–29
Chance's fracture of L1. (A) Anterior wedging of anterior body with horizontal fracture through the posterior elements. (B) Frontal view reveals a fracture involving the laminae and spinous process of L1. (C) Coned-down view shows vertebral body involvement.

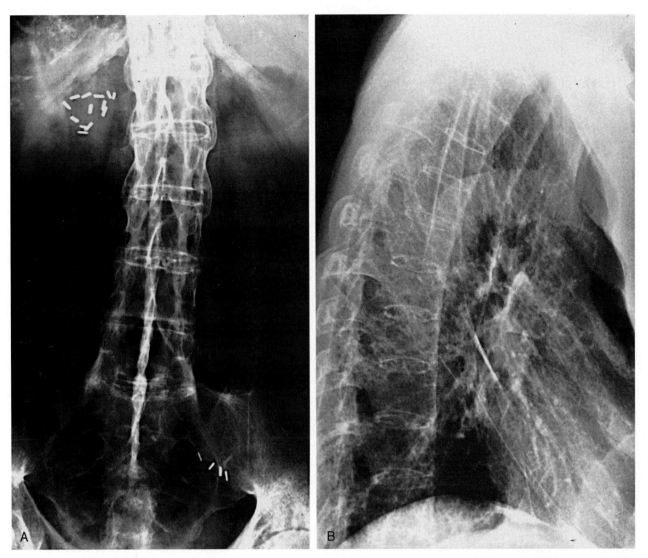

Figure 4–30

Ankylosing spondylitis. Complete ankylosis of sacroiliac joints on (A) frontal and (B) lateral views. Vertical line density is consistent with ossification of posterior ligaments and syndesmophyte formation.

REFERENCES

1. Pope TL Jr, Riddervold HO: Spine. *In* Keats TE (ed): Emergency Radiology, 2nd ed. Chicago: Year Book, 1989.

2. Turetsky DB, Vines FS, et al: Technique and use of supine oblique views in acute cervical spine trauma. Ann Emerg Med 1993;22:685–689.

3. Freemyer B, Knopp R, et al: Comparison of five-view and three-view cervical spine series in the evaluation of patients with cervical trauma. Ann Emerg Med 1989;18:818–821.

4. Macdonald RL, Schwartz ML, et al: Diagnosis of cervical spine injury in motor vehicle crash victims: How many x-rays are enough? J Trauma 1990;30:392–397.

5. Young JWR, Mirvis SE: Cervical spine trauma. *In* Mirvis SE, Young JWR (eds): Imaging in Trauma and Critical Care. Baltimore: Williams & Wilkins, 1992.

6. Stiell IG, Wells GA, et al: Variation in emergency department use of cervical spine radiography for alert, stable trauma patients. Can Med Assoc J 1997;156(11):1537–1544.

7. Zabel DD, Tinkoff G, et al: Adequacy and efficacy of lateral cervical spine radiography in alert, high-risk blunt trauma patients. J Trauma 1997;43(6):952–958.

8. Velmahos GC, Theodorou D, et al: Radiographic cervical spine evaluation in the alert asymptomatic blunt trauma victim: Much ado about nothing? J Trauma 1996;40(5):768–774.

9. Miller MO, Gehweiler JA, et al: Significant new observations on cervical spine trauma. AJR 1978;130:659–663.

10. Samuels LE, Kerstein MD: Routine radiologic evaluation of the thoracolumbar spine in blunt trauma patients: A reappraisal. J Trauma 1993;34(1):85–89.

11. Meldon SE, Moettus LN: Thoracolumbar spine fractures: Clinical presentation and the effect of altered sensorium in major injury. J Trauma 1995;39(6):1110–1114.

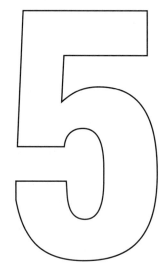

Pelvic and Lower Extremity Radiography

GARY A. JOHNSON, MD

PELVIS

The pelvic ring comprises bilateral iliac, ischial, and pubic bones and the sacrum. The ring has three joints: the bilateral sacroiliac joints and the pubic symphysis. Thus it is not a single bone but rather three bony elements supported by interosseous ligaments. The majority of the soft tissue stresses are supported in the sacroiliac joints. The pubic symphysis stabilizes the pelvic ring anteriorly but does not provide a significant amount of vertical strength.

Stable fractures of the pelvis are often described as those that do *not* compromise the weight-bearing function of the pelvis. Such injuries include pubic fractures, avulsion fractures, and acetabular fractures. Pubic and ischial ramus fractures (Fig. 5–1) are common and can be unilateral or bilateral.

Avulsion fractures include fractures of the iliac crest, anterior superior iliac spine, and anterior inferior iliac spine. These injuries often affect young athletes. The iliac crest is a site of attachment for numerous muscles, including the tensor fasciae latae, transverse abdominal muscles, gluteus medius, and external oblique abdominal muscles. Avulsion of the anterior superior iliac spine is relatively common. A typical mechanism of injury is forceful contraction of the sartorius muscle, which commonly occurs in sprinters. The anterior inferior iliac spine

may be avulsed by contraction of the rectus femoris muscle. This may happen to runners or athletes who kick.[1]

Unstable fractures of the pelvic ring involve the posterior aspects of the pelvis and result from powerful forces. The mechanism of injury is often used to describe pelvic fractures. A lateral compression mechanism (as when a car strikes a pedestrian from the side) may cause pubic ramus fractures, compression fractures of the sacrum, fractures of the iliac wing, or rupture of the sacroiliac joint (Fig. 5–2). A second mechanism is anteroposterior compression. These injuries may include diastasis of the symphysis pubis (Fig. 5–3) or of the sacroiliac joint or posterior and lateral sacroiliac dislocation. Forceful AP compression may cause the hemipelvis to rotate outward and opens the pelvis like a book (Fig. 5–4). Such AP compressions are associated with severe vascular injury and high morbidity and mortality rates.[2] Even a small amount of movement in the sacroiliac joint, without bone injury, can result in significant hemorrhage (Fig. 5–5).

A third mechanism of injury is vertical shear like that imparted in a fall from a height onto an extended leg. Such fractures are usually associated with a vertical fracture of the iliac crest (Fig. 5–6), dislocation of a sacroiliac joint, and vertical displacement of the iliac fragment. Several mechanisms of injury may occur simultaneously, and a combination of these injuries may occur.

Text continued on page 144

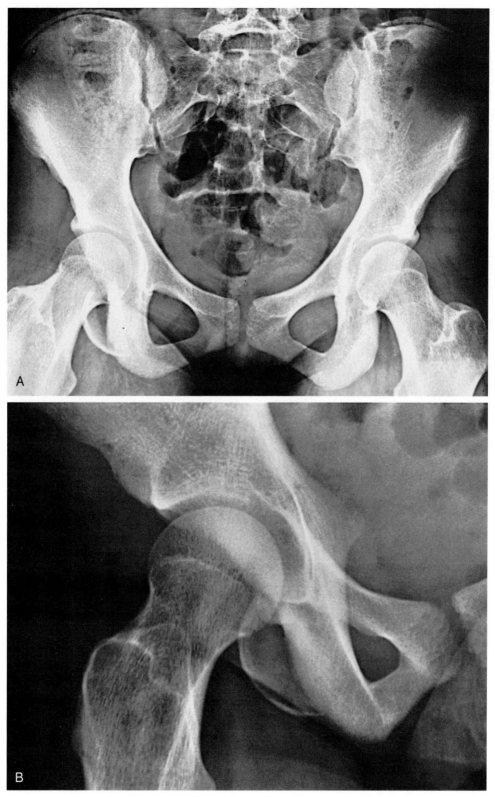

Figure 5–1
Ischial tuberosity avulsion fracture, (A) *frontal and* (B) *oblique views.*

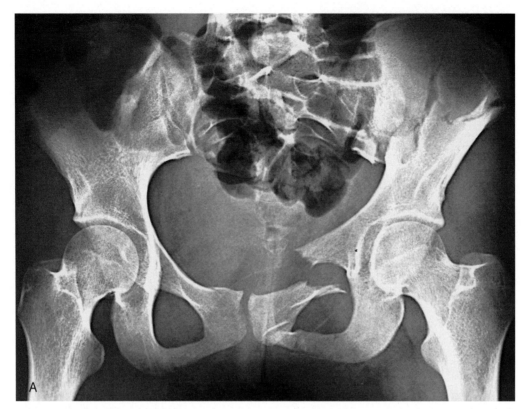

Figure 5–2
Comminuted left iliac wing fracture, left superior and inferior pubic rami, and right symphysis pubis fractures seen on frontal view (A).

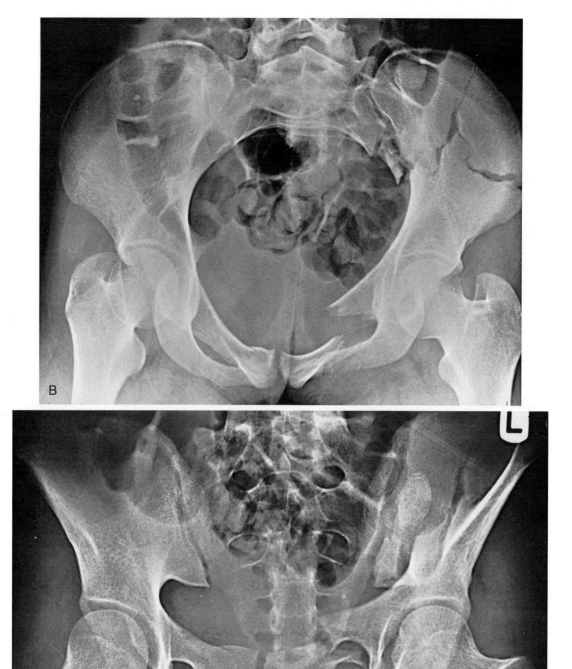

Figure 5–2 *Continued*
(B) *Inlet and* (C) *outlet views help to evaluate pelvic fracture further.*

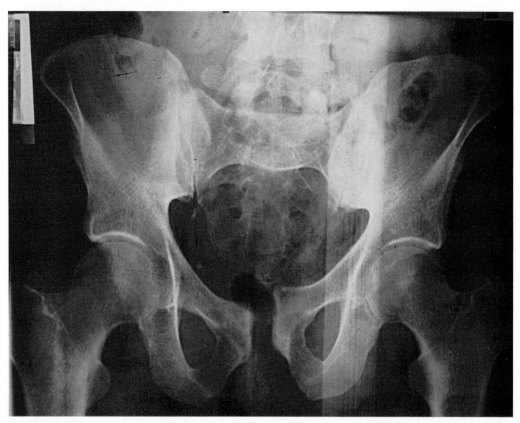

Figure 5–3
Pubic symphysis disruption. The pubic symphysis and the right sacroiliac joint both show widening. A small avulsion fracture may also be present at inferior aspect of the right sacroiliac joint.

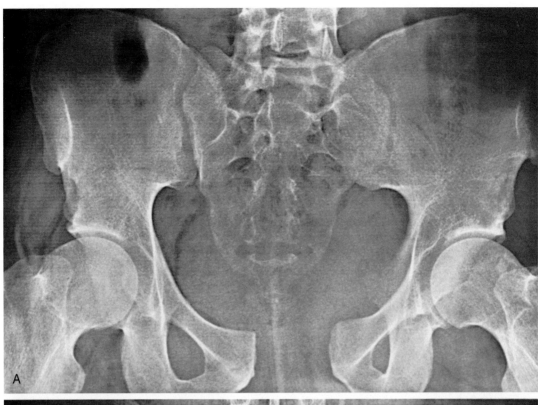

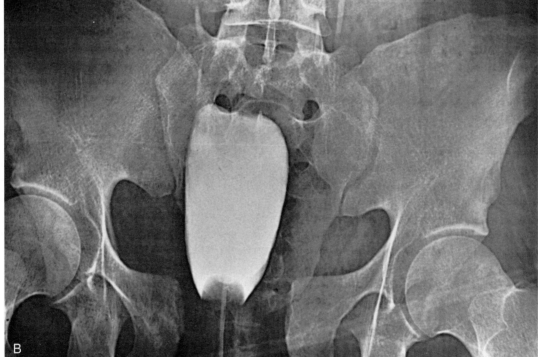

Figure 5–4

(A) "Open-book" injury with pubic symphysis diastasis and sacroiliac joint widening. Increase in soft tissue density in pelvis is compatible with hematoma. (B) Cystogram demonstrates pear-shaped bladder secondary to pelvic hematoma.

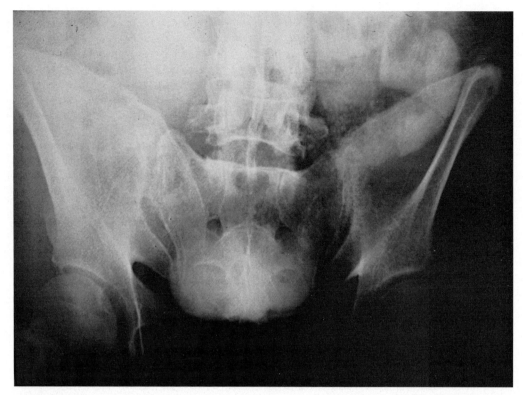

Figure 5–5
Sacroiliac joint disruption demonstrated with intravenous contrast medium. The bladder is elevated secondary to pelvic hematoma. The right sacroiliac joint is widened. No bone injury is present.

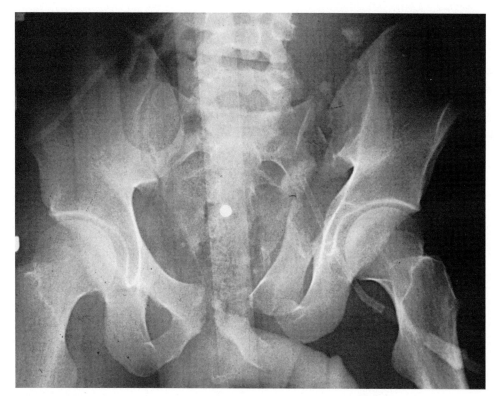

Figure 5–6

Vertical shear injury of the left iliac wing: disruption and vertical displacement of the left iliac bone, sacroiliac joint disruption, and left pubic fracture. Diastasis of the symphysis pubis is present. An intravenous catheter is seen in the left groin.

ACETABULUM

The acetabulum is formed by the ilium and the pubic and ischial bones. It is frequently described as having an anterior and a posterior column. The posterior column includes the roof and bears most of the weight. The posterior rim is the part of the acetabulum most often fractured. Ossicles may form around the acetabulum and can be confused with fractures (Fig. 5–7). Transverse fractures can be simple or complex (Fig. 5–8). The routine AP pelvis film and oblique projections (Judet's view) may help to demonstrate them. Plain radiography is generally inadequate to fully delineate acetabular fractures, and CT is recommended.

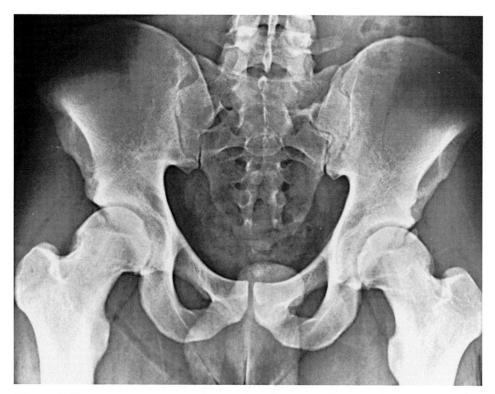

Figure 5–7
Well-defined bone ossicles of both acetabula compatible with ununited secondary ossification centers.

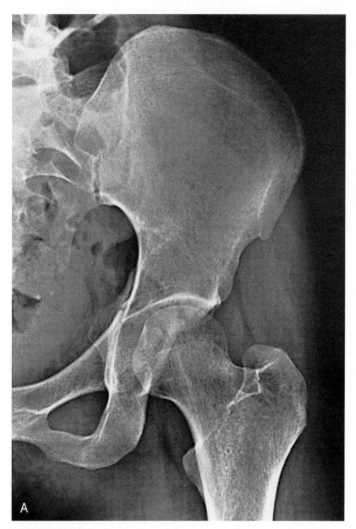

Figure 5–8
Minimally displaced transverse acetabular fracture, (A) frontal and (B) frog-leg views.

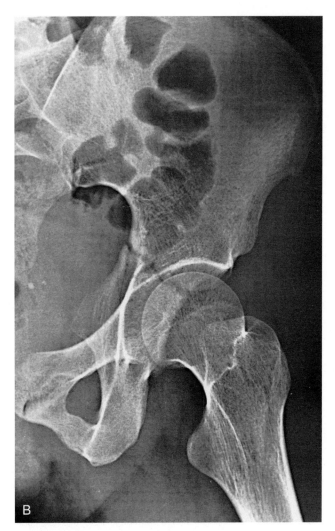

Figure 5–8 *Continued*

HIP

The hip can be dislocated by a high-energy injury. Posterior dislocations are the most common hip dislocations (Figs. 5–9, 5–10). The mechanism is most often transmission of a force along the long axis of the femur when the hip is flexed. An auto deceleration may force a passenger's leg into the dashboard and dislocate the hip. Anterior dislocations are much less common but may result from a fall with the leg extended at the hip or with the hip abducted. A dislocation that pushes the femoral head into the obturator fossa is called an "obturator dislocation" (Fig. 5–11). Hip dislocations may be complicated by avascular necrosis of the femoral head or neurovascular injury. Fracture of the acetabulum or femoral head is also common with hip dislocation.

Hip fractures are most common in patients older than 50 years. The vast majority are the result of simple falls in patients with osteoporosis. Fractures through the femoral neck are common. Displaced fractures are often complicated by osteonecrosis and nonunion. Patients with impacted femoral neck fractures (Fig. 5–12) may still be ambulatory and may even have referred pain in the lower abdomen, groin, or knee.

A fracture line that extends from the greater to the lesser trochanter is often termed "intertrochanteric." Such fractures typically are comminuted and have several fragments. Muscle insertions onto the lesser trochanter (psoas muscle) or the greater trochanter (gluteal muscles) may cause distraction of the fracture fragments (Figs. 5–13, 5–14).

Fractures distal to the lesser trochanter are often called "subtrochanteric." They can be extensions of intertrochanteric fractures or isolated subtrochanteric injuries. Typically, they have a cantilevered configuration with a large angle in relation to the proximal femur (Fig. 5–15).

Disruption of the vascular supply to the hip may cause avascular necrosis (Fig. 5–16). This is seen radiographically as sclerosis and flattening of the hip. Fracturing the midshaft of the femur requires great force. These fractures are generally easily seen once the proper radiograph is obtained (Fig. 5–17).

Text continued on page 158

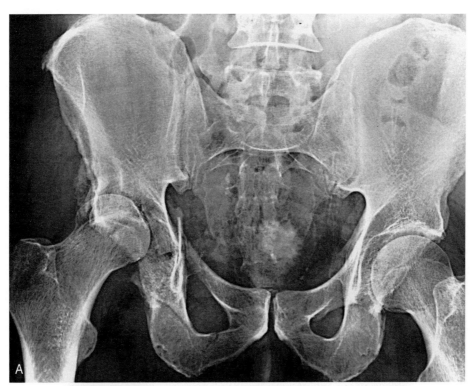

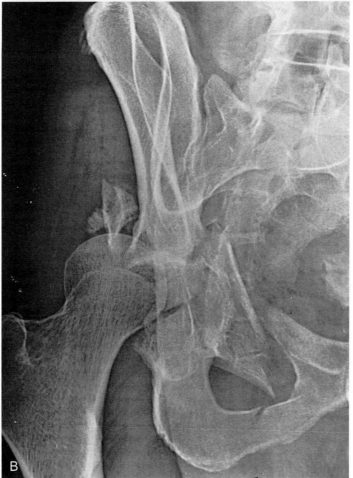

Figure 5–9

(A) *Posterior fracture-dislocation of right hip.* (B) *Dislocation on Judet's view. Comminuted fracture of acetabulum and fractures of superior and inferior pubic rami are also demonstrated.*

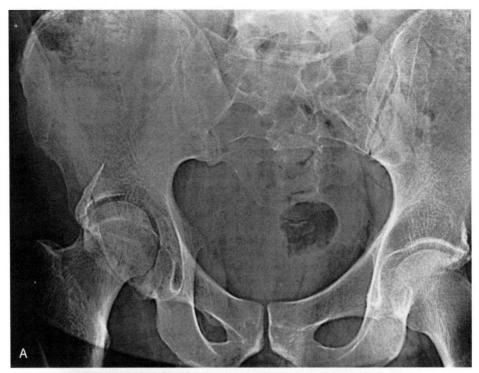

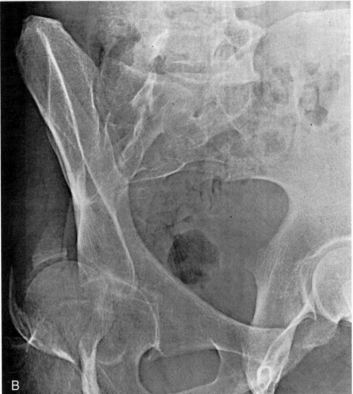

Figure 5–10
Posterior fracture-dislocation of right hip with posterior acetabular lip fracture, (A) AP and (B) Judet's views.

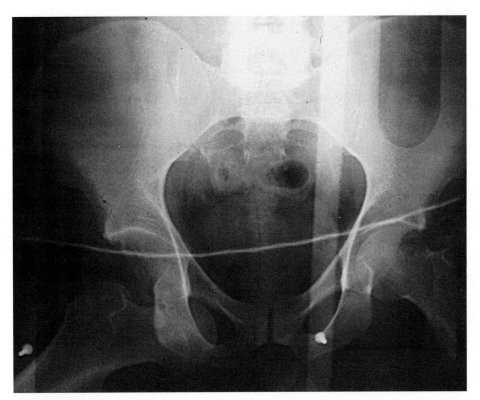

Figure 5–11
Obturator dislocation of the right hip. The right femoral head is seen in the obturator fossa.

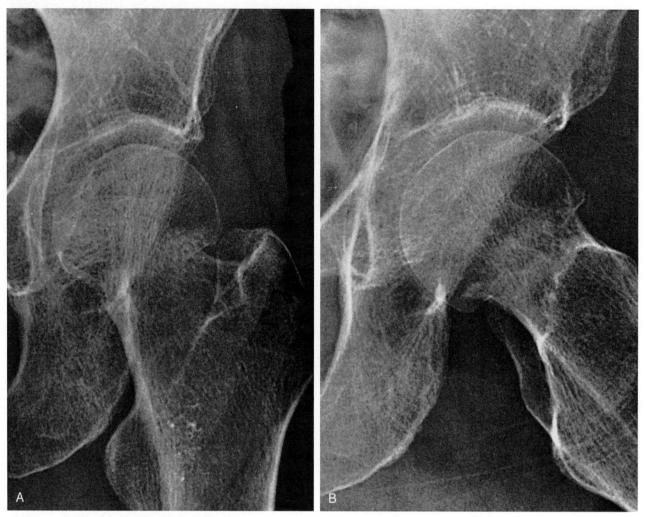

Figure 5–12
Impacted femoral neck (subcapital) fracture of proximal femur, (A) *frontal and* (B) *frog-leg views.*

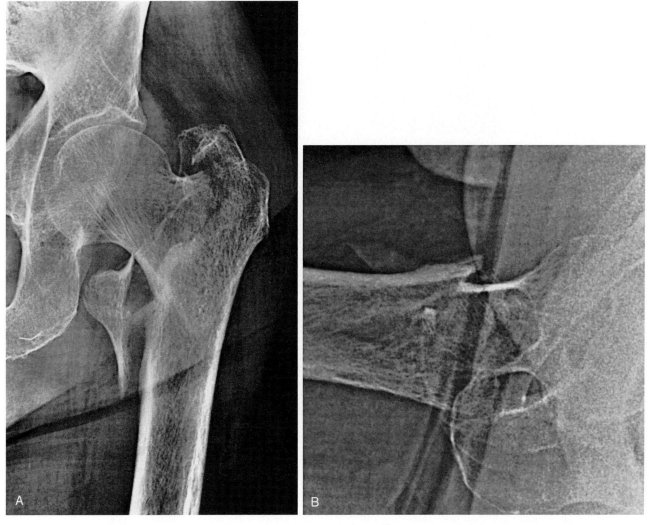

Figure 5–13
(A) *Frontal and* (B) *cross-table lateral views demonstrate intertrochanteric fractures.*

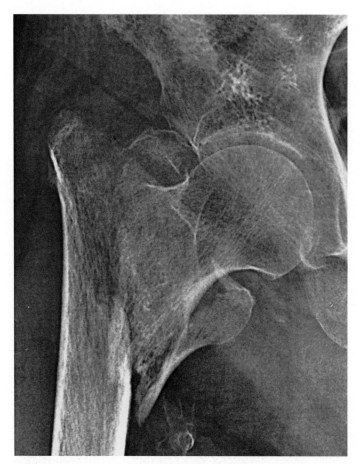

Figure 5-14
Comminuted (four-part) intertrochanteric fracture.

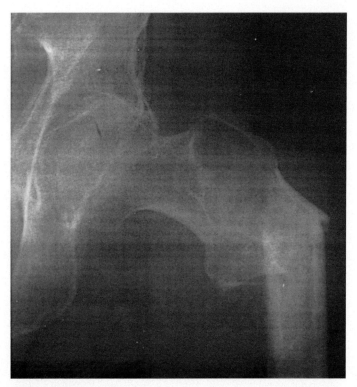

Figure 5–15
Subtrochanteric fracture with marked angular deformity.

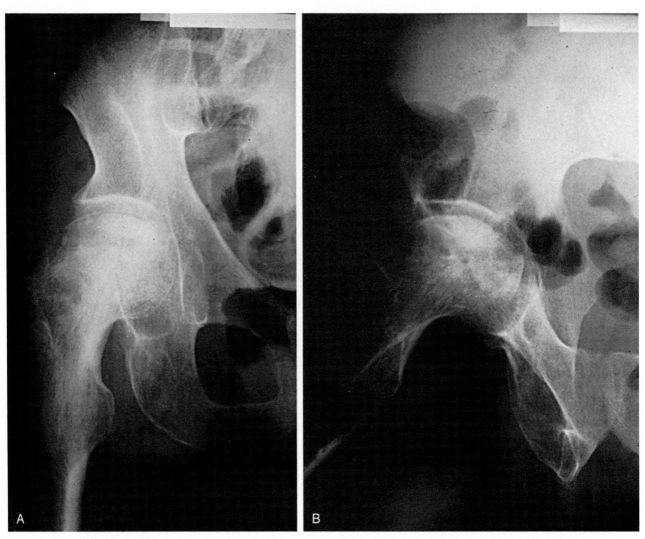

Figure 5–16
Avascular necrosis of the right femoral head on (A) *frontal and* (B) *oblique views. Femoral head is flattened and bone is sclerotic.*

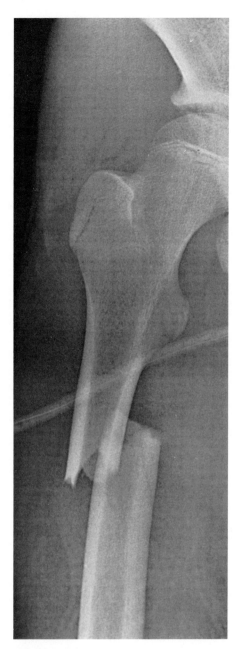

Figure 5–17
Transverse fracture at the junction of the proximal and middle thirds of the femur.

KNEE

A knee injury may be manifested as principally a bone injury or as a soft tissue injury with associated bone findings. The extensor mechanism of the knee includes the patella. Patellar fractures may be difficult to visualize on frontal views (Fig. 5–18). Lateral, oblique, or sunrise (Merchant's) views may be helpful (Fig. 5–19). A knee joint effusion may be visible on the lateral radiograph (Figs. 5–20, 5–21). It will appear as a fluid density exerting mass effect on the surrounding tissue. A lipohemarthrosis implies that a fracture has allowed intramedullary fat into the joint.

Avulsion fractures around the femoral tibial articulation may suggest soft tissue injury. An avulsion fracture of the lateral tibia at the insertion site of the joint capsule is referred to as Segond's fracture (Fig. 5–22). A tear of the medial collateral ligament of the knee may have some ectopic calcification. If it is visible on plain films, it is known as Pellegrini-Stieda disease (Fig. 5–23). Avulsions of either condylar eminence may indicate disruption of

an anterior cruciate or a posterior cruciate ligament (Fig. 5–24).

A force transmitted along the long axis of the tibia may injure the articular surface of the tibia. These fractures are called "tibial plateau fractures." These may be subtle on plain films, and careful inspection of the plateau (especially the lateral aspect) is advisable. A knee effusion should be present (Fig. 5–25).

A complete disruption of the ligamentous structures of the knee may result in dislocation of the femoral tibial articulation (Fig. 5–26). These injuries generally require great force and are associated with neurovascular injuries. Soft tissue calcification may also be seen (Fig. 5–27).

Tibial shaft fractures are high-energy injuries (Fig. 5–28) and are usually clinically obvious. Owing to the proximity of the epidermis and bone, these fractures may be open. The fibula generally bears no weight, and a fracture may go undetected (Fig. 5–29). Injuries to the proximal fibula are associated with the injuries to the recurrent peroneal nerve and may result in foot drop (Fig. 5–30).

Text continued on page 172

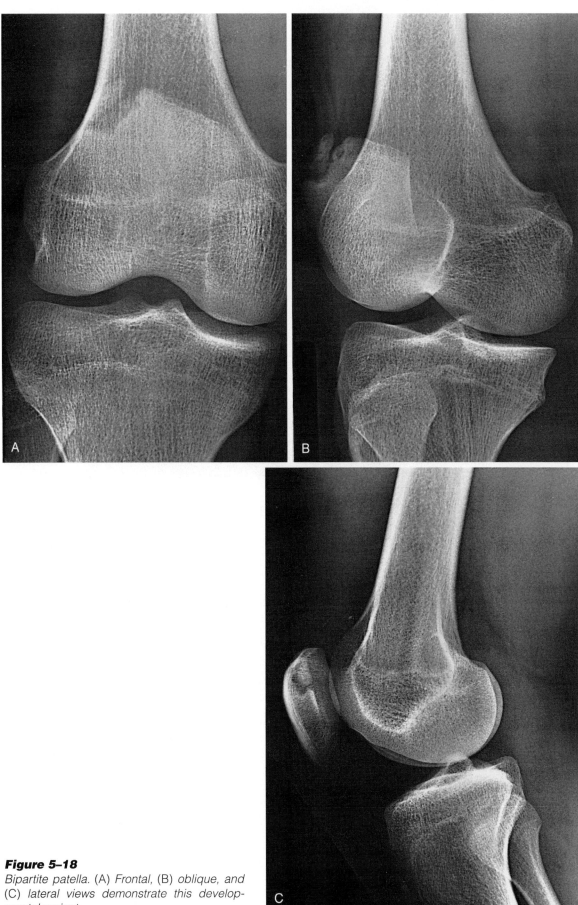

Figure 5–18
Bipartite patella. (A) Frontal, (B) oblique, and (C) lateral views demonstrate this developmental variant.

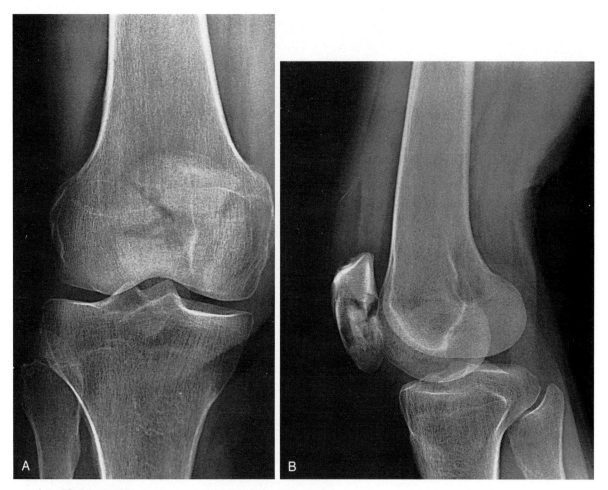

Figure 5–19
Stellate fracture of the patella with lipohemarthrosis (fat-fluid level), (A) AP and (B) lateral views.

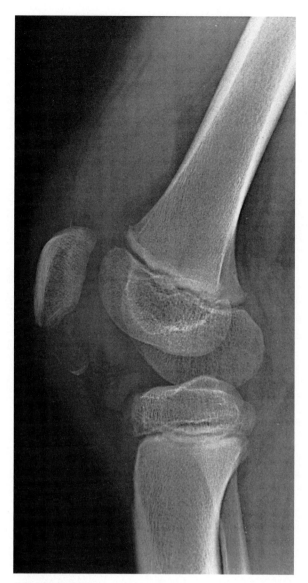

Figure 5–20
Avulsion fracture of the inferior pole of the patella with large joint effusion.

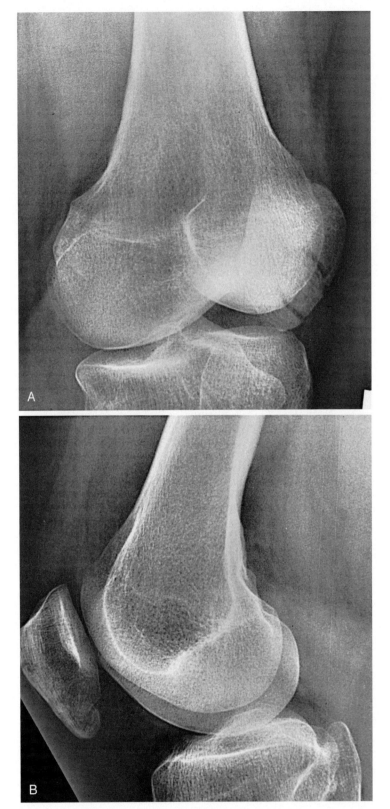

Figure 5–21
Patellar fracture of the middle and inferior pole is best seen on the oblique view (A). (B) *Lateral and* (C) *Merchant's (sunrise) views.*

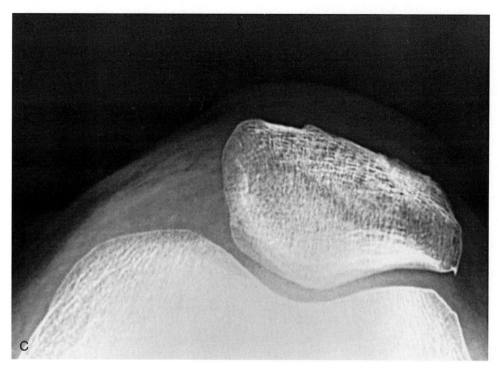

Figure 5–21 *Continued*

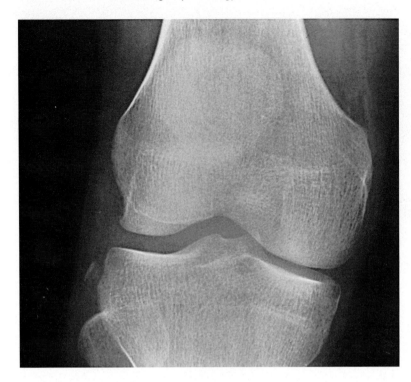

Figure 5–22
Segond's fracture. Bone fragment adjacent to the proximal lateral tibia is characteristic of an avulsion fracture of the tibia at the site of attachment of the lateral capsular ligament. This finding is often associated with anterior cruciate ligament tears and meniscal injuries.

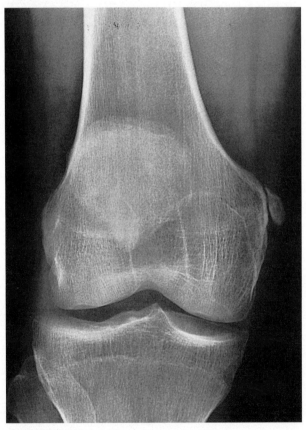

Figure 5–23
Pellegrini-Stieda disease. Calcification in the soft tissues adjacent to the medial femoral condyle is secondary to chronic medial collateral ligament injury.

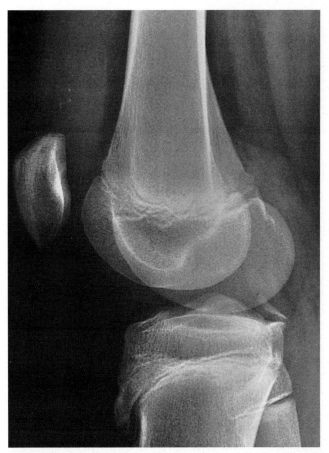

Figure 5–24
*Avulsion fracture of the posterior tibial plateau secondary to
a posterior cruciate ligament injury. A large joint effusion is
also present.*

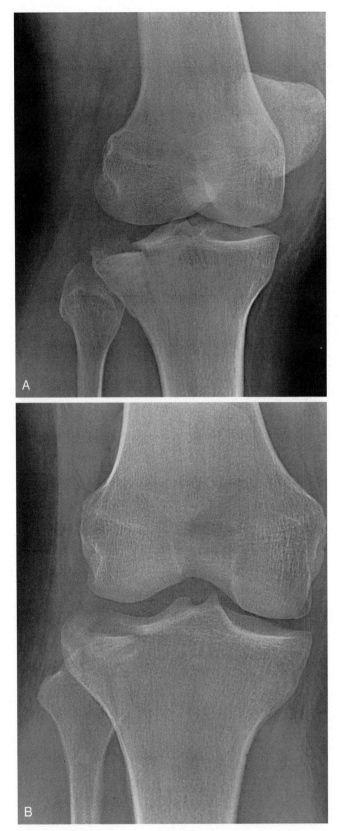

Figure 5–25
Depressed lateral tibial plateau fracture with lipohemarthrosis, (A) oblique, (B) frontal, and (C) lateral views.

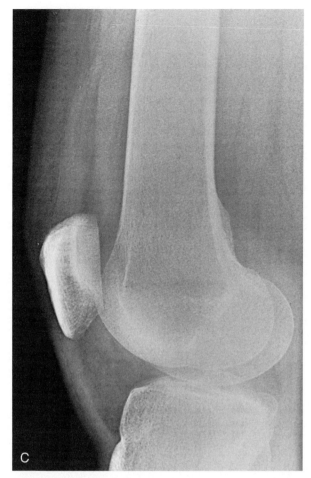

Figure 5–25 *Continued*

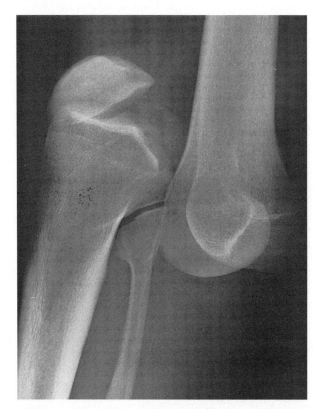

Figure 5–26
Posterior knee dislocation, lateral view.

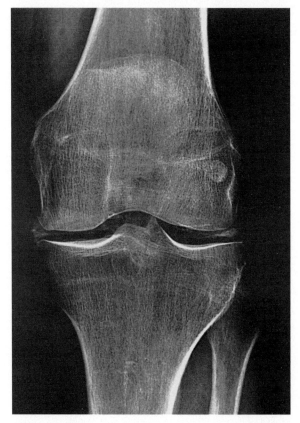

Figure 5–27
Chondrocalcinosis. Calcification of the medial and lateral menisci.

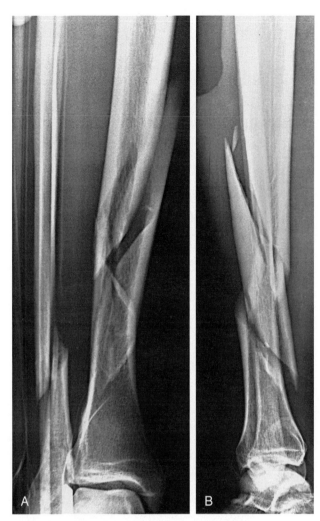

Figure 5-28
Spiral fracture of the distal tibia and oblique fracture of the distal fibula, (A) frontal and (B) lateral views.

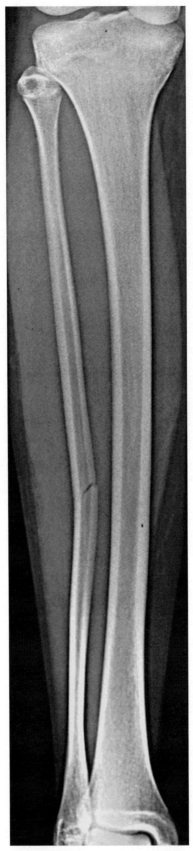

Figure 5–29
Midshaft fibular fracture. This view demonstrates bowing and an incomplete (greenstick) fracture.

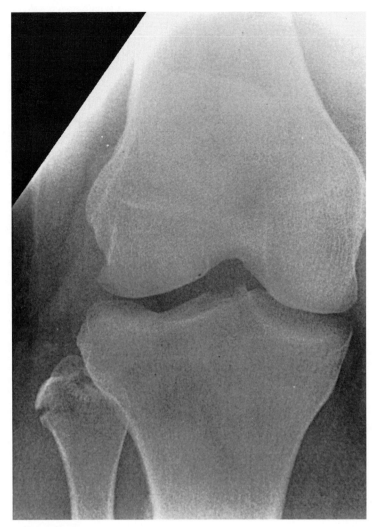

Figure 5–30
Fracture of the fibular head.

ANKLE

The ankle is made up of the distal tibia, fibula, and talus. The joint is supported by the syndesmosis between the tibia and fibula and by ligaments between the fibula and the talus and calcaneus and the deltoid ligament between the tibia and the talus and calcaneus. The talus has no direct muscle insertions and, therefore, serves as a mechanical conduit between the leg and foot.

Most ankle injuries are caused by abnormal rotational movement. Inversion of the foot (adduction) stretches the lateral malleolus and its ligaments. This may produce a lateral ankle sprain or a fracture of the distal fibula or proximal fifth metatarsal (Figs. 5–31, 5–32). Forceful ankle loading in inversion causes the talus to transmit the force to the medial malleolus and may fracture the distal tibia (Fig. 5–33).

An injury with the foot in relative plantar flexion will disrupt the syndesmosis and displace the talus posteriorly. This may injure the posterior malleolus (posterior aspect of the tibia; Figs. 5–34 through 5–36).

Eversion of the foot (abduction) will disrupt the deltoid ligament and the medial malleolus. The talus will move laterally and disrupt the syndesmosis (Fig. 5–37). A powerful force will cause the talus to dislocate laterally and injure the distal fibula.

A fall from a height with the foot in midposition produces pure vertical loading on the ankle. This may cause a pilon fracture. The talus is driven into the tibia and the articular surface, and the tibial shaft is comminuted. Typically, the medial and the posterior malleolus are broken and the ligaments are disrupted.

Maisonneuve's fracture (Fig. 5–38) is a distal fibular fracture in combination with disruption of the syndesmosis and a proximal fibular fracture and is frequently associated with injury to the recurrent peroneal nerve. Ankle injuries have been classified in a number of ways—by mechanism of injury, anatomic site, and relation of the fracture to the level of the tibial articular surface. In fact, ankle fractures often defy these classifications.

Utility of diagnostic radiography has been debated in the literature. The Ottawa ankle rules have been advanced as a method for clinically screening patients for radiography. Stiell and associates[3, 4] studied these guidelines and have shown that applying them can be cost-effective without limiting clinical yield.

Text continued on page 180

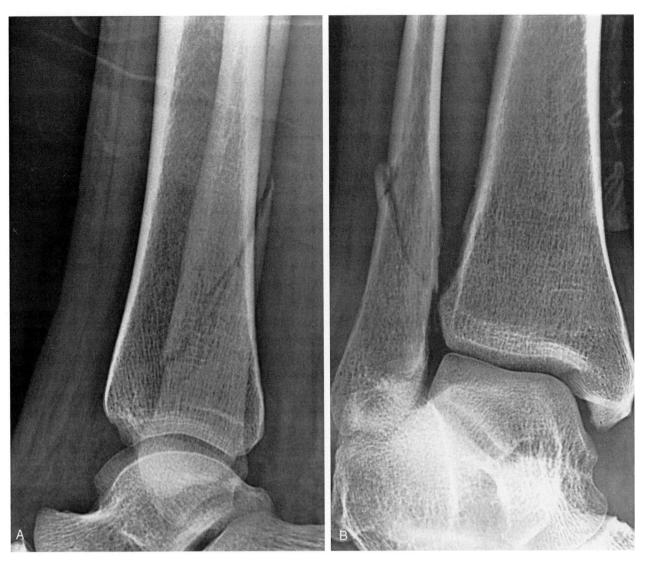

Figure 5–31
Oblique fracture of distal fibula, (A) lateral and (B) frontal views. The ankle mortise is intact.

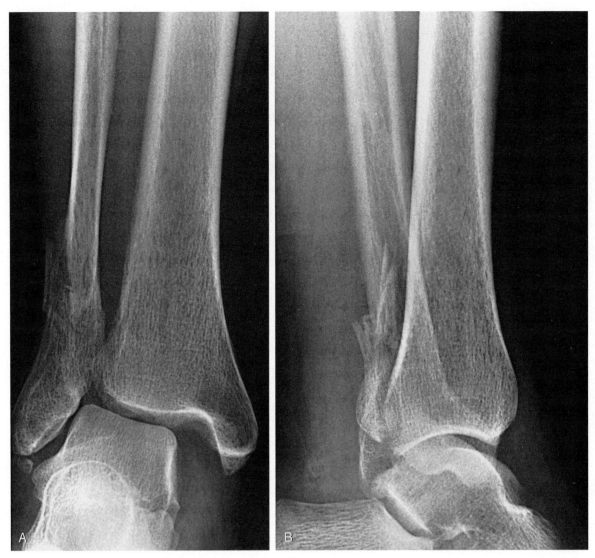

Figure 5–32
Oblique fracture of the fibula with lateral displacement of the talus, (A) AP and (B) lateral views. Medial joint space widening secondary to deltoid ligament rupture. The distal tibia is also fractured posteriorly.

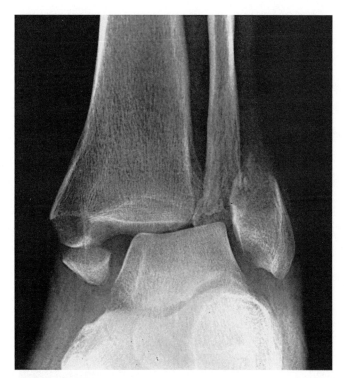

Figure 5–33
Bimalleolar fracture. Transverse fracture of the medial malleolus and oblique fracture of distal fibula with lateral displacement of the talus.

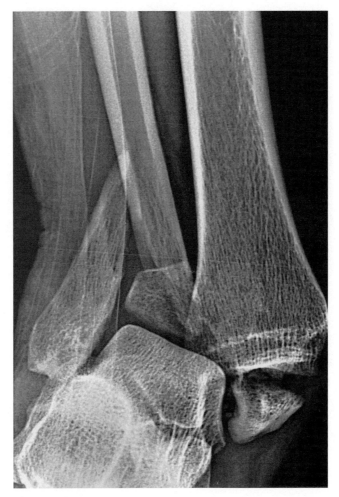

Figure 5–34
Trimalleolar fracture. Transverse fracture of the medial malleolus, oblique fracture of the distal fibula, and posterolateral displacement of the talus with fracture of the distal tibia posteriorly.

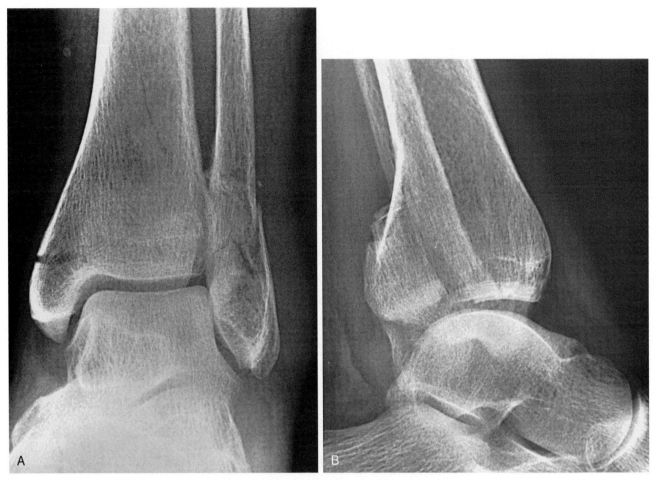

Figure 5–35
Trimalleolar fracture, (A) frontal and (B) lateral views. Transverse nondisplaced fracture of the medial malleolus. Comminuted oblique fracture of the distal fibula and fracture of posterior aspect of the distal tibia.

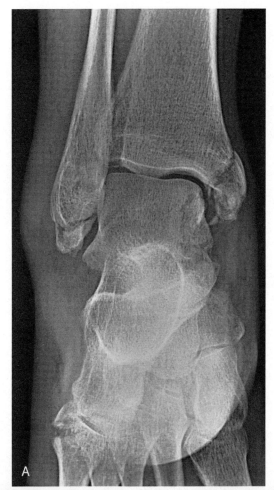

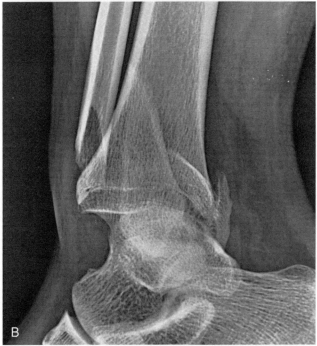

Figure 5–36
Multiple fractures. Bimalleolar, talus, navicular, and base of the fifth metatarsal fractures, (A) frontal and (B) lateral views.

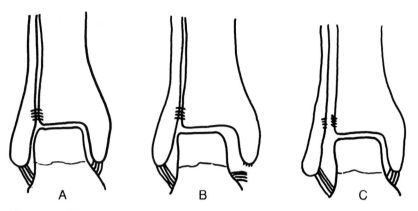

Figure 5–37
Ankle. (A) Normal mortise, (B) widened medial joint, and (C) syndesmotic disruption with widening between the tibia and fibula. (Miller MD: Commonly missed orthopedic problems. Emerg Med Clin North Am 1992; 10:151.)

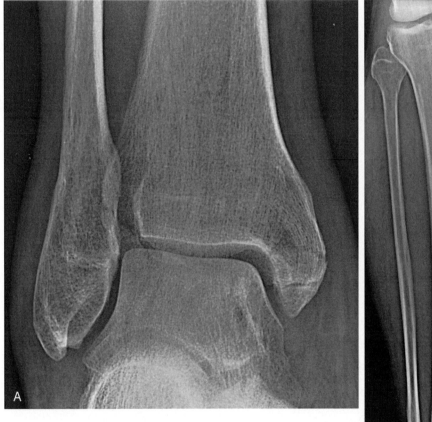

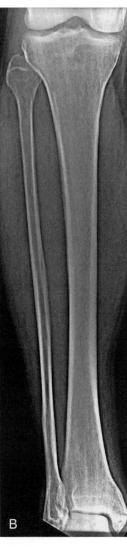

Figure 5–38
Maisonneuve's fracture, (A) AP ankle and (B) frontal tibiofibular views. There is a nondisplaced fracture of the proximal fibula and a transverse fracture of the medial malleolus. The lateral aspect of the distal tibia is also fractured.

FOOT

Forcing the talus against the tibia may cause an osteochondral fracture (osteochondritis dissecans; Figs. 5–39, 5–40). Loading of the foot and dorsal hyperflexion may transmit a force through the neck of the talus. Hawkin's classification recognizes three types of vertical talar neck fractures: type I, nondisplaced; type II, subluxation of the subtalar joint, and type III, dislocation of the subtalar and ankle joints.

Falls from a height may cause a calcaneal fracture. These are often associated with lumbar spine fractures. Boehler's angle (Fig. 5–41) has been used to identify more subtle calcaneus fractures (Figs. 5–42 through 5–44). The calcaneus has a superior peak in its midsection and an anterior and a posterior lip. On a lateral view, the superior aspect of the calcaneus roughly describes a W. Lines drawn from the peak to the anterior and posterior pinnacles form the angle called "Boehler's angle." A normal value is 28 to 40 degrees.

Normal adolescent calcaneal epiphysis may have a sclerotic appearance (Fig. 5–45). Plantar fasciitis may result in a bone spur at the calcaneal insertion site (Fig. 5–46).

The most common foot fracture is that of the base of the fifth metatarsal, an injury typically caused by an inversion injury that transmits a tensile load to the bone. Fracture of the metaphysis of the fifth metatarsal is Jones' fracture (Fig. 5–47), whereas avulsion of the base of the metatarsal (the tuberosity) is not Jones' fracture (Fig. 5–48). Because, in earlier texts, this fracture was defined incorrectly, an anatomic description of the injury is preferable to the eponym.

Vertical compression of the foot commonly causes metatarsal fractures (Figs. 5–49 through 5–51). The midfoot (tarsus) and the metatarsals constitute Lisfranc's joint. Great force applied to Lisfranc's joint may cause a fracture-dislocation. Typically, all of the metatarsals are dislocated laterally (a homolateral dislocation; Fig. 5–52). The dislocation is divergent when the second through the fifth metatarsals are dislocated laterally and the first metatarsal is dislocated immediately. A fracture of the base of the second metatarsal typically occurs at its ligamentous insertion to the cuneiforms. Freiberg's infarction may be manifested as sclerosis of the second metatarsal head (Fig. 5–53).

Stress fractures are commonly in the lower extremities. Initial radiographs are unremarkable, but follow-up films reveal fracture healing (Figs. 5–54 through 5–56). Radiographs will demonstrate radiopaque foreign bodies (Fig. 5–57). Charcot's joint may develop in the foot or ankle (Fig. 5–58).

Text continued on page 200

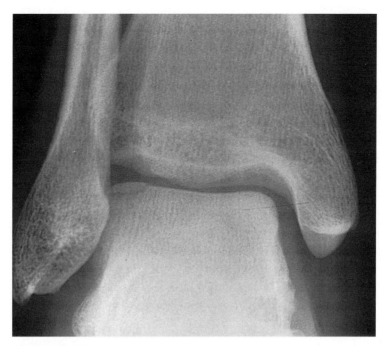

Figure 5–39
Osteochondral fracture on the lateral aspect of the dome of the talus.

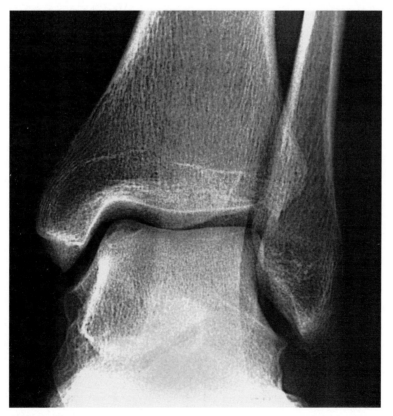

Figure 5–40
Osteochondritis dissecans of the talus. A small osteochondral defect of the medial dome of the talus.

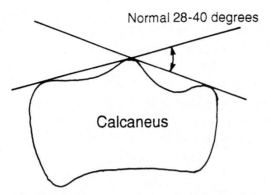

Figure 5–41
Boehler's angle. Boehler's angle is calculated on lateral foot radiographs by drawing intersecting lines as illustrated here. The normal Boehler's angle measures 28 to 40 degrees. Abnormal measurements are very suggestive of calcaneal fracture. (Miller MD: Commonly missed orthopedic problems. Emerg Med Clin North Am 1992; 10:151.)

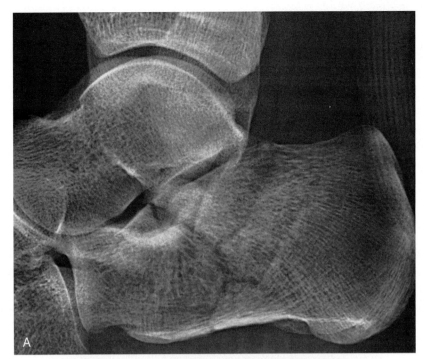

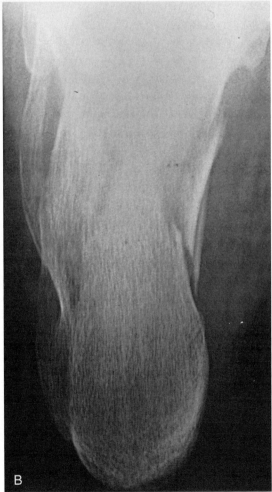

Figure 5–42
Comminuted calcaneus fracture with involvement of the subtalar joint and resultant decrease in the Boehler's angle, (A) lateral and (B) axial views.

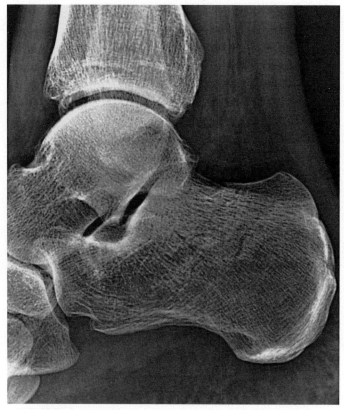

Figure 5–43
Calcaneal fracture. Subtle fracture is seen in the body of the calcaneus. There is cortical disruption of the superior aspect of the calcaneus posterior to the talus.

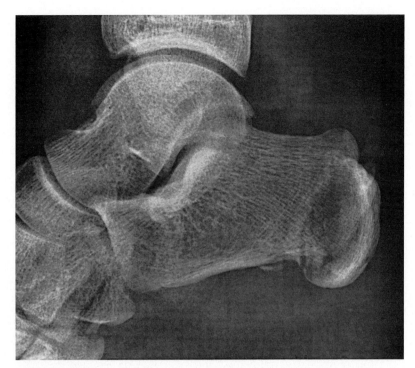

Figure 5–44
Fracture of the calcaneus and cuboid bones, lateral view.

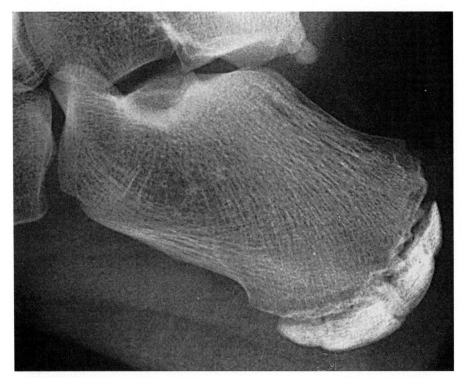

Figure 5–45
Normal variation in the appearance of the calcaneus in an adolescent.

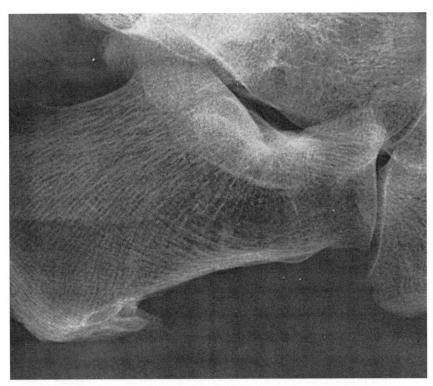

Figure 5–46
Calcaneal spur at the insertion of the plantar fascia.

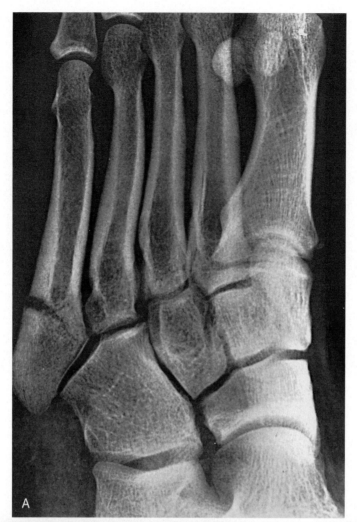

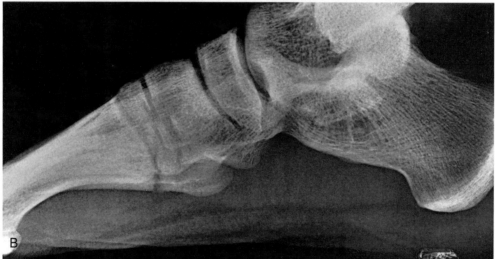

Figure 5–47
Jones' fracture (metaphyseal fracture of the fifth metatarsal). (A) Oblique and (B) lateral views show transverse fracture just distal to the tuberosity. Jones' fracture should not be confused with fractures of the tuberosity.

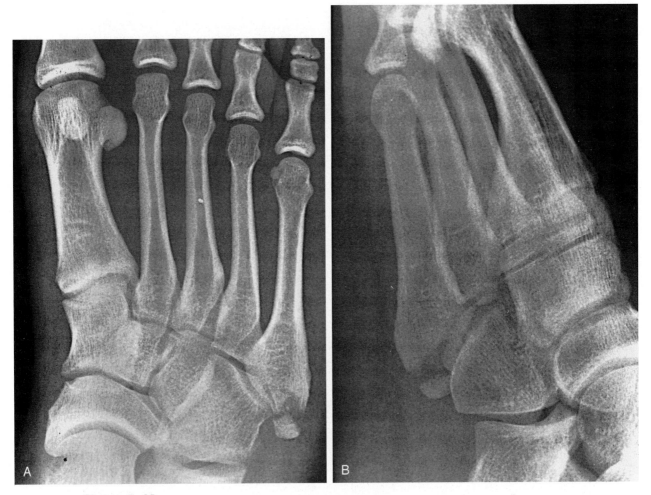

Figure 5–48
Avulsion fracture of the tuberosity of the base of the fifth metatarsal, (A) frontal and (B) lateral views. (Not Jones' fracture).

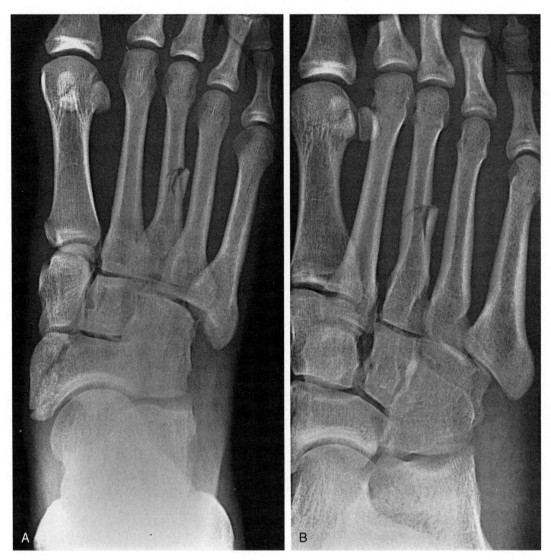

Figure 5–49
Fracture of midshaft of the third metatarsal and medial aspect of the navicula, (A) frontal and (B) oblique views. Lateral subluxation of the fourth and fifth metatarsals with respect to the cuboid.

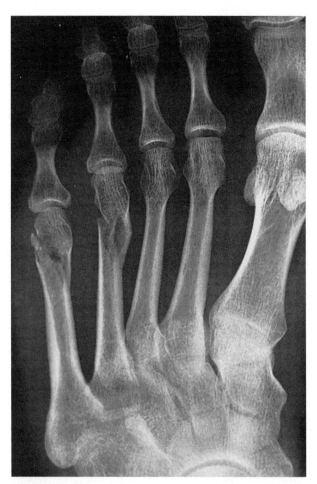

Figure 5–50
Fracture of the metatarsal necks of the fourth and fifth digits.

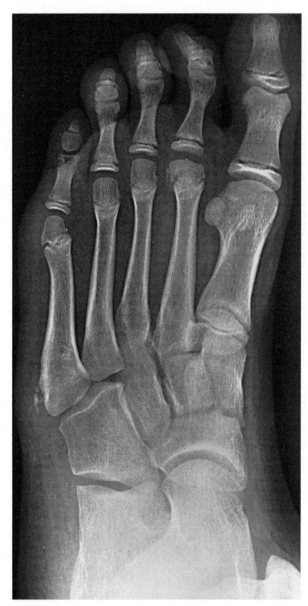

Figure 5–51
Fracture of the epiphysis of the second metatarsal. A secondary ossification center at the base of the fifth metatarsal is not a fracture.

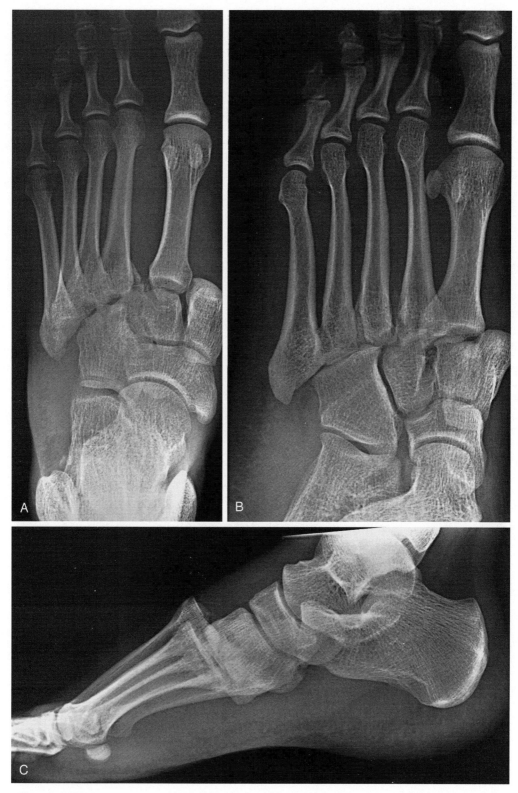

Figure 5–52

Homolateral Lisfranc's fracture-dislocation, (A) frontal, (B) oblique, and (C) lateral views. Avulsion of the base of the second metatarsal and lateral dislocation of the second through the fifth metatarsals. The first metatarsal is also dislocated laterally.

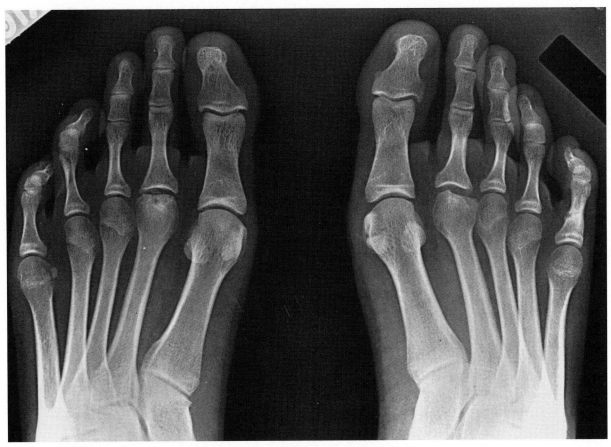

Figure 5–53
Bilateral Freiberg's infarction. Flattening of the second metatarsal heads bilaterally is present. Increased incidence in women may be related to high-heeled shoes. There is also a stress fracture of the proximal phalanx of the right fifth digit.

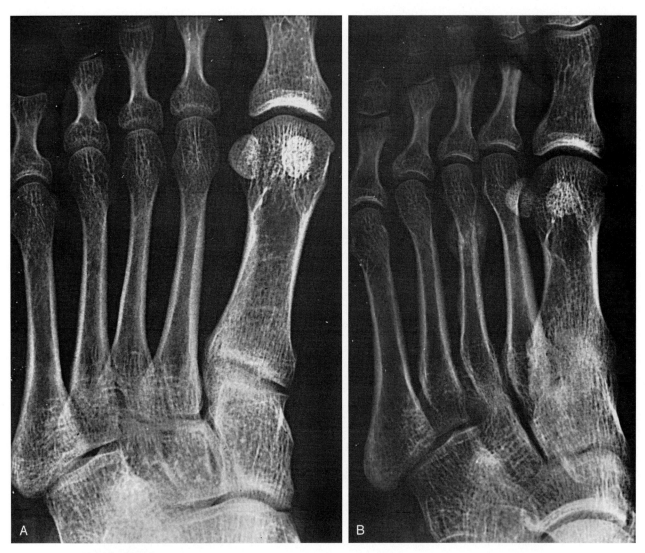

Figure 5–54
Stress fracture of the third metatarsal. (A) Initial film demonstrated no fracture. (B) Follow-up image reveals prominent callus formation about subtle fracture line.

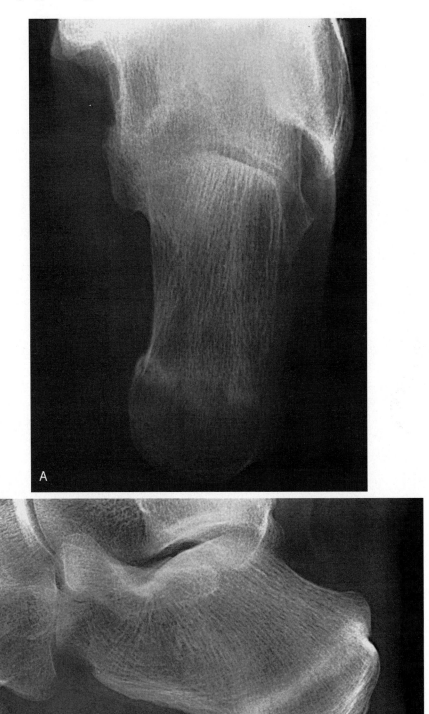

Figure 5–55
Stress fracture of the calcaneus, (A) axial and (B) lateral views.

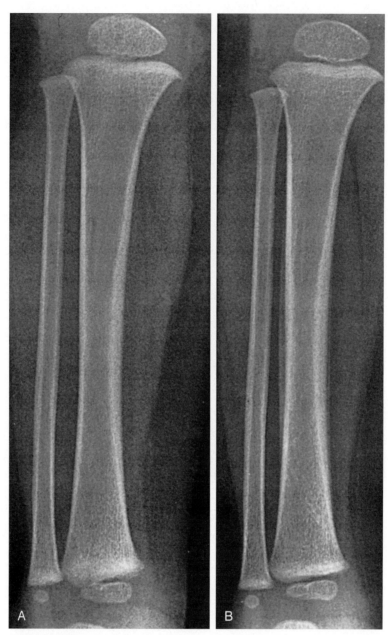

Figure 5–56
Periosteal reaction. (A) Initial radiograph was negative; however, (B) follow-up radiographs after a week demonstrated periosteal reaction about midshaft of tibia that most likely is related to radiographically occult fracture.

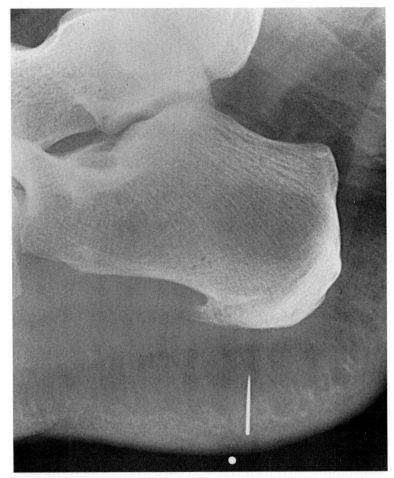

Figure 5–57
Soft tissue foreign body. Metallic foreign body is seen in the soft tissue below the calcaneus. Round radiopaque skin marker overlies the foreign body.

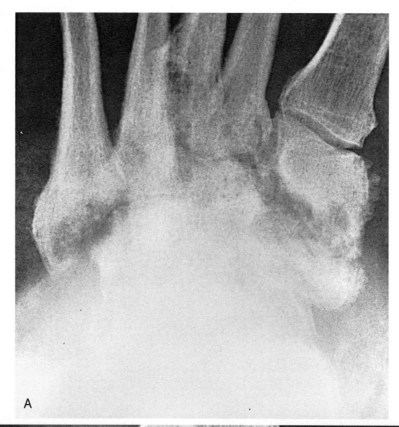

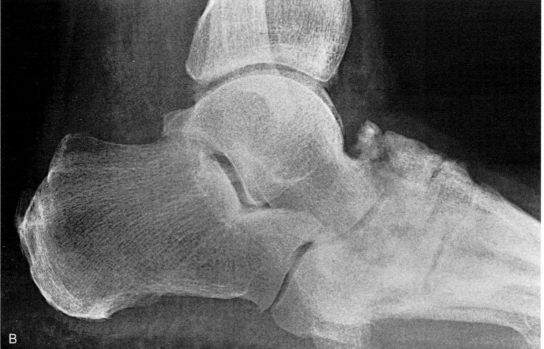

Figure 5–58
Charcot's joint, (A) *frontal and* (B) *lateral views. Diabetic patient had marked deformity and destruction about the tarsometatarsal joints.*

REFERENCES

1. Paletta GA, Andrish JT: Injuries about the hip and pelvis in the young athlete. Clin Sports Med 1995;14(3):591–628.

2. Alonso JE, Lee J, et al: The management of complex orthopedic injuries. Surg Clin North Am 1996;76(4):879–903.

3. Stiell IG, McKnight RD, et al: Implementation of the Ottawa Ankle Rules. JAMA 1994;271:827–832.

4. Stiell I, Wells G, et al: Multicentre trial to introduce the Ottawa ankle rules for use of radiography in acute ankle injuries. Br Med J 1995;311(7005):594–597.

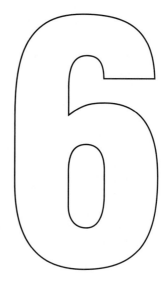

Upper Extremity Radiography

GARY A. JOHNSON, MD

SHOULDER

The human shoulder has great range of motion—at the expense of stability. Glenohumeral ligaments and the rotator muscle cuff support the shoulder. Typically, glenohumeral dislocation is anterior and inferior. Often, it is the result of a fall on an arm that is both abducted and externally rotated. The humerus can then lever against the acromion and be dislocated. Patients with inherently unstable shoulders may suffer a dislocation from a direct blow, typically one from behind.

Radiographic confirmation of a shoulder dislocation requires visualizing the glenohumeral joint. AP and oblique shoulder films may suggest dislocation, but they cannot adequately rule it out. An axillary radiograph obtained with the x-ray tube directed up into the axial and the radiographic plate placed behind the shoulder should clearly demonstrate the glenohumeral joint. In patients who cannot abduct the shoulder, a transscapular Y view may confirm that the humeral head no longer articulates with the glenoid (Fig. 6–1).

Posterior shoulder dislocations are often more difficult to assess radiologically. An AP film may appear normal or show excessive space between the glenoid fossa and the humeral head. An axillary or Y view will show the posterior dislocation.

Shoulder dislocations may cause impaction of fractures of the humeral head. A Hill-Sachs lesion, depression of the posterolateral aspect of the humeral head, is typically caused by inferior dislocation that caused it to strike the glenoid. A tear of the labrum may produce an avulsion fracture of the anterior glenoid, a lesion called "Bankart's fracture" (see Fig. 6–1).

A fall onto an adducted shoulder may result in an acromioclavicular joint separation. A grade I separation describes stretched, but not disrupted, ligaments; grade II, with torn acromioclavicular ligaments; and grade III, disruption of both acromioclavicular and coracoclavicular ligaments (Fig. 6–2).

A fall on an adducted shoulder can also fracture the clavicle (Fig. 6–3), typically in the middle third of the bone. Proximal clavicular injuries ought to raise suspicion of intrathoracic injury. Similarly, proximal humerus fracture can result from a fall onto an adducted shoulder (Figs. 6–4, 6–5).

The scapula may be fractured by a direct blow or may suffer an avulsion from a muscle contraction (Fig. 6–6). Generally, a great force is required to fracture the scapula with a direct blow.

Soft tissue calcifications may be associated with arthritis (Fig. 6–7) or tendinitis (Fig. 6–8).

Text continued on page 212

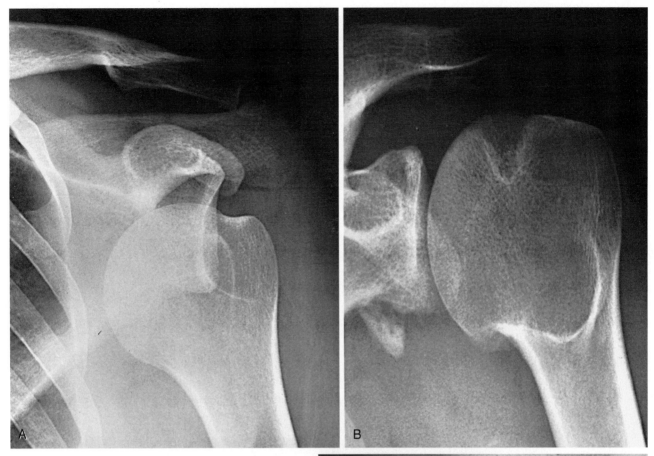

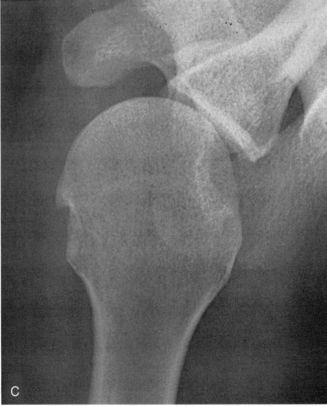

Figure 6–1
Anterior shoulder dislocation. (A) A subcoracoid anterior dislocation as seen on oblique (Grashey's) view. (B) Postreduction axillary view shows good alignment with humoral head and glenoid fossa. A Hill-Sachs defect is clearly seen. (C) An apical oblique view reveals Hill-Sachs deformity and Bankart's fracture of the inferior glenoid rim.

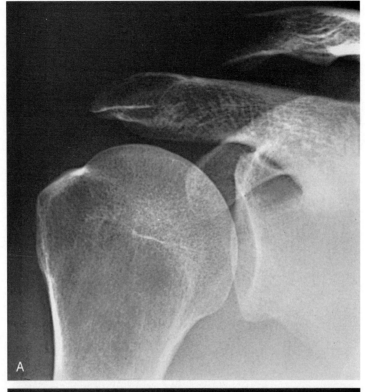

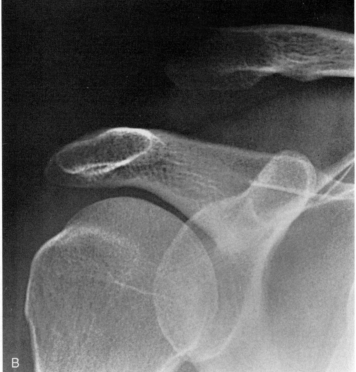

Figure 6–2
Acromioclavicular joint injury. Widened acromioclavicular joint and coracoacromial distance indicate a type III injury. Two films of same patient obtained (A) 2 years before the injury and (B) after it.

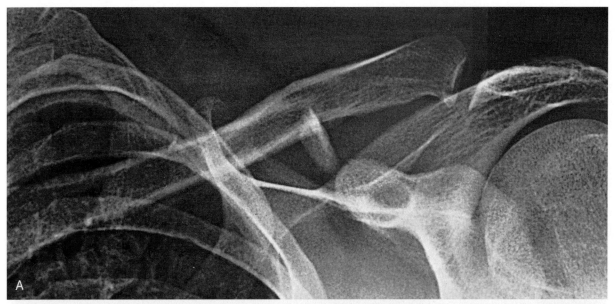

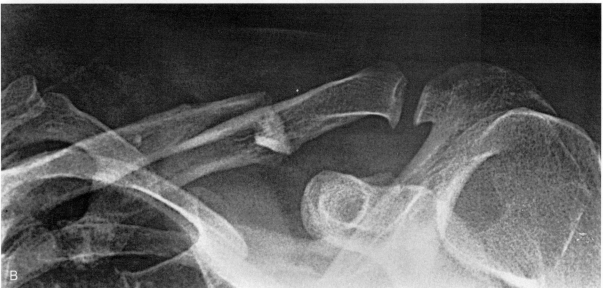

Figure 6–3

Two views of a clavicular fracture. (A) Initial radiograph shows a bone fragment between coracoid and clavicle, but no fracture line. (B) An angled view shows a clavicular fracture in the middle third of the bone. An inferior spur at the acromioclavicular joint is consistent with arthritic change.

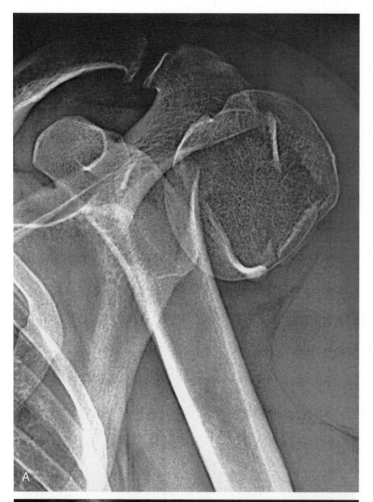

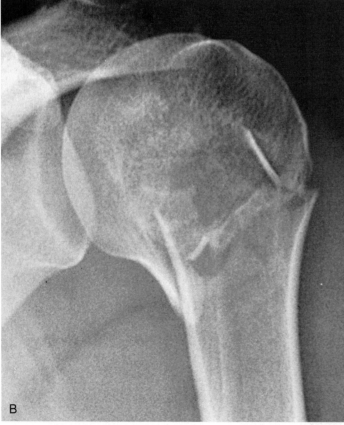

Figure 6–4
Comminuted displaced surgical neck fracture. (A)
Original AP view shows marked displacement of hu-
meral head. (B, C) Postreduction views show marked
improvement in position and alignment with an intact
glenohumeral relationship.

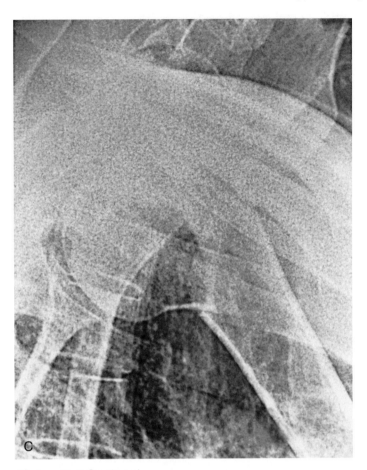

Figure 6–4 *Continued*

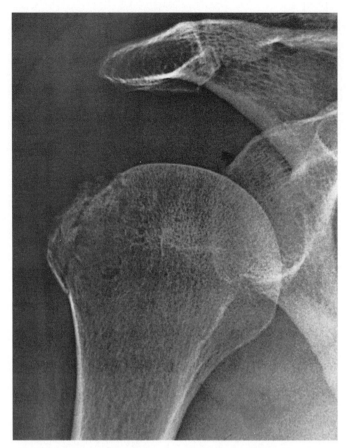

Figure 6–5
*Fracture of greater tuberosity of the humerus. The humeral
head is displaced inferiorly, a finding that may represent subluxation or pseudosubluxation (from hematoma formation).*

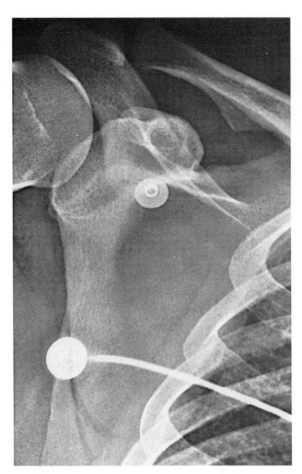

Figure 6–6
Comminuted fracture of the inferior aspect of the scapula.

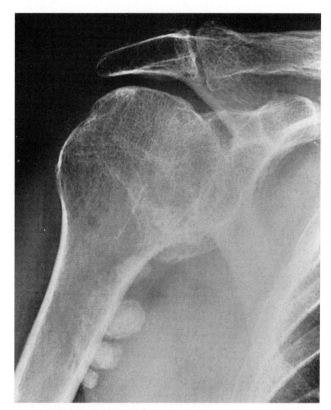

Figure 6–7
Loose bodies around the proximal humerus with arthritic changes of the glenohumeral joint. Spurring of the acromioclavicular joint is shown.

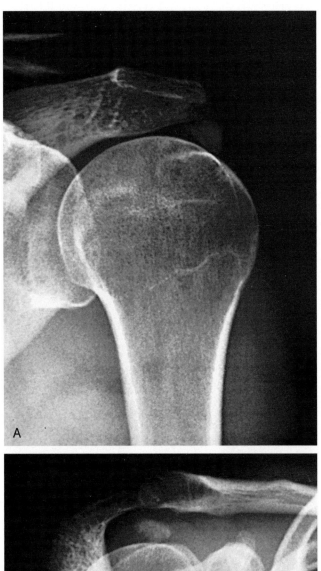

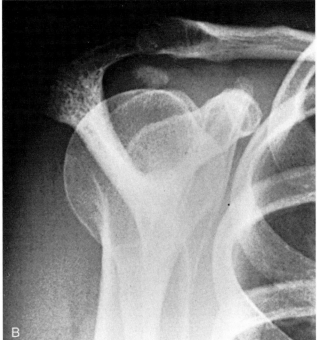

Figure 6–8
Calcific tendinitis. A dense, homogeneous calcification is visible superior to the humeral head. Adjacent bone is intact. (A) AP and (B) outlet views.

ELBOW

A direct fall on the olecranon process is often the mechanism of olecranon fracture (Fig. 6–9). The olecranon may also be avulsed by contraction of the triceps muscle. In adults, the most common elbow fracture is a radial head fracture, an injury that is often the result of a fall on an outstretched arm. Radial head fractures can be occult. Such injuries manifested only by an elbow effusion, which is identified radiographically by an anterior or posterior "sail sign." In children, an occult fracture of the elbow is most likely a supracondylar fracture of the humerus. Visualization of the posterior joint capsule (posterior sail sign) should always be con-

sidered abnormal. To produce the anterior sail sign, the normal fat pad must be pushed up and away from the humerus in which position it has the shape of a triangular sail (Figs. 6–10, 6–11). Radial head fractures are best visualized on an oblique view that is coned down on the radial head (Fig. 6–12).

Dislocations of the humeroulnar joint may result from a fall on the outstretched arm. Typically, the radius is dislocated from both the ulna and the humerus (Fig. 6–13). A fracture (typically of the ulna) may be associated with the dislocation.

Intracondylar fractures of the humerus often have a T or Y configuration. Comminution of the fragments is also common. Neurovascular injury is a serious concern with both elbow dislocations and intracondylar humeral fractures (see Fig. 6–13).

Text continued on page 218

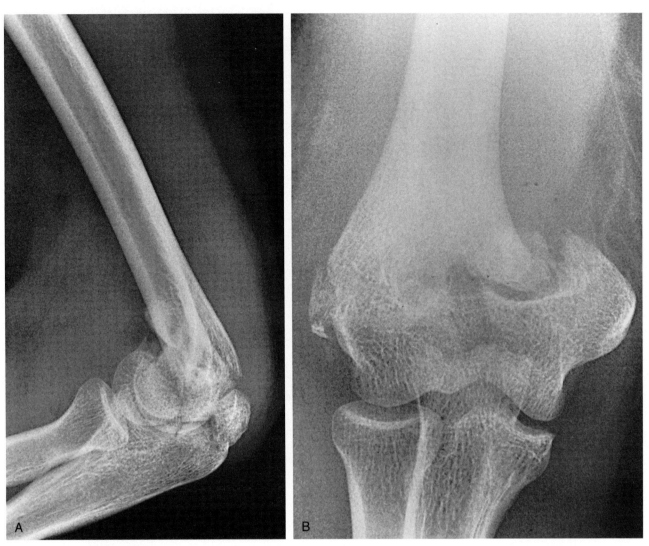

Figure 6–9
(A) *AP and* (B) *lateral views of a comminuted supracondylar fracture and an olecranon process fracture.*

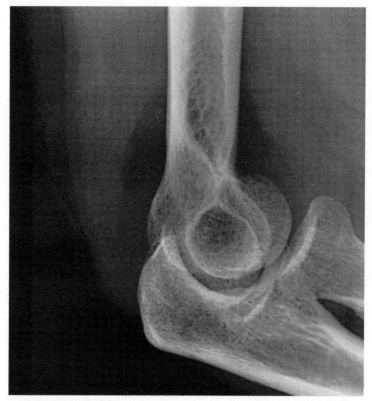

Figure 6–10
Large anterior sail sign and posterior fat pad sign compatible with joint effusion. No fractures are radiographically apparent, although these findings are suggestive of an occult fracture.

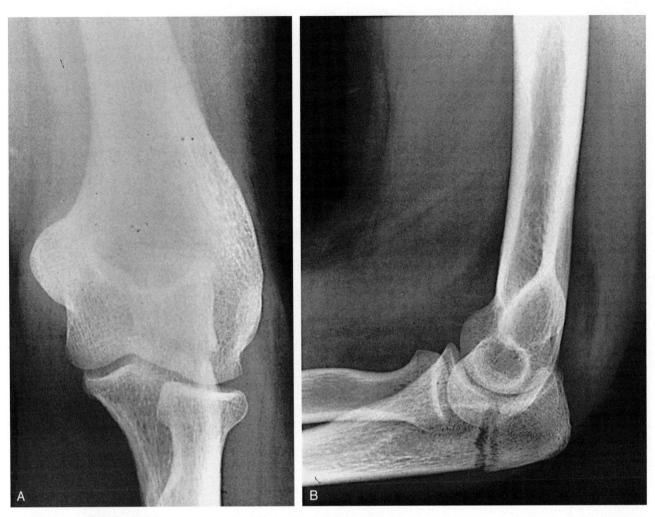

Figure 6–11
(A) *Frontal and* (B) *lateral views of intraarticular proximal ulnar fracture. Anterior sail sign and posterior fat pad sign are compatible with joint effusion.*

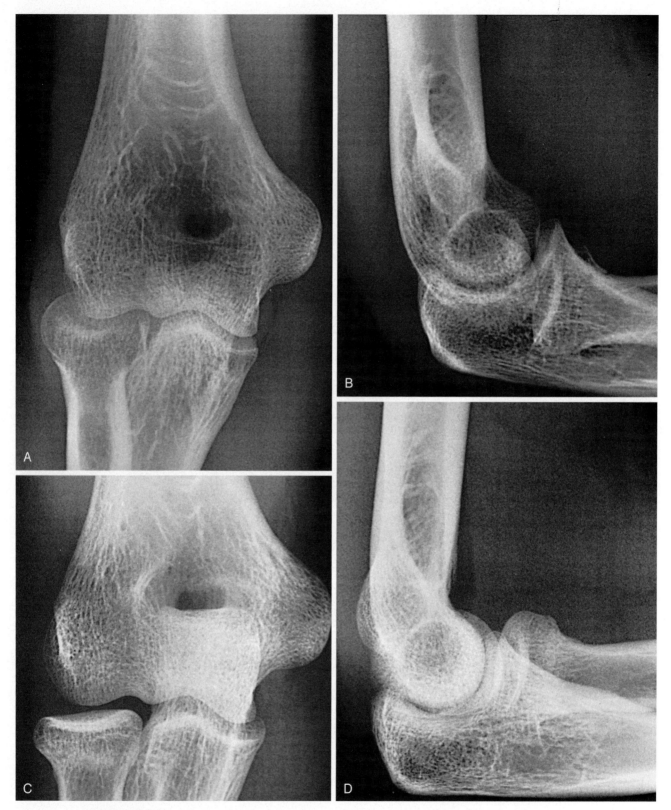

Figure 6–12

Radial neck fracture. (A) Frontal view shows slight cortical disruption at the radial neck. (B) Posterior and anterior fat pads are visible, which findings indicate a joint effusion. Radial neck cortical lucency is visible. (C, D) Follow-up films reveal decreasing joint effusion and increased sclerosis compatible with interval healing.

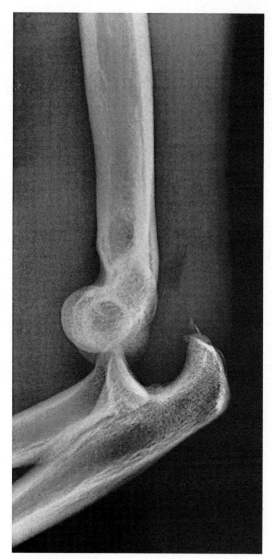

Figure 6–13
Posterior dislocation of the elbow. The ulna is displaced posteriorly with respect to the humerus. There is a small fracture fragment adjacent to the olecranon process.

FOREARM

Fractures of the distal radius generally result from a fall on an outstretched arm. A distal radial fracture with volar angulation is commonly called "Smith's fracture" (Fig. 6–14); a transverse radial fracture with dorsal angulation, "Colles' fracture" (Fig. 6–15). In these fractures, the radial articular surface is intact. An ulnar styloid fracture frequently accompanies Smith's or Colles' fracture.

A fall on an outstretched arm may transmit enough force through the lunate to fracture the articular surface of the distal radius. Typically, such breaks produce three fragments. The radial styloid is avulsed and a medial dorsal fragment is also present. Commonly, the distal radioulnar joint at the wrist is dislocated.

Forearm fractures of the ulna can occur alone or with fractures of the radius. An isolated fracture of the ulna may result from direct force ("nightstick fracture"; Fig. 6–16). Most fractures of the forearm involve both bones. Galeazzi's fracture is a distal radius fracture (classically at the junction of the middle and distal thirds) with dislocation of the distal radioulnar joint. Monteggia's fracture is a break in the midshaft of the ulna with radial head dislocation (Fig. 6–17). A fracture of either the radius or the ulna should always raise suspicion of dislocation of the distal radioulnar joint or the proximal radiohumeral joint.

Text continued on page 224

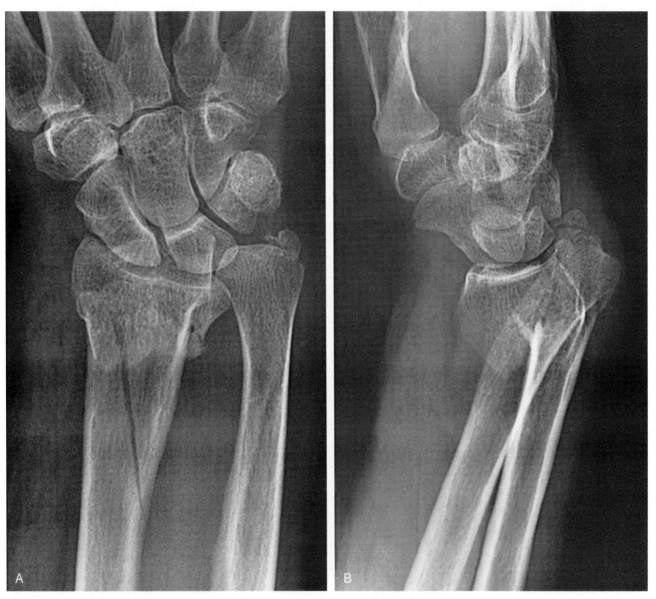

Figure 6–14
Smith's fracture, (A) frontal and (B) lateral views. Comminuted fracture of the distal radius with volar displacement and angulation. Ulnar styloid fracture is also present.

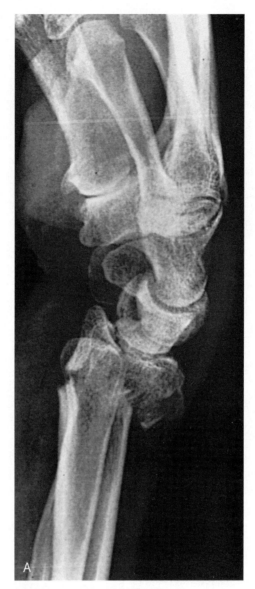

Figure 6–15
*Colles' fracture with intraarticular extension,
(A) lateral and (B) frontal views. The distal
radius fragment is dorsally displaced.*

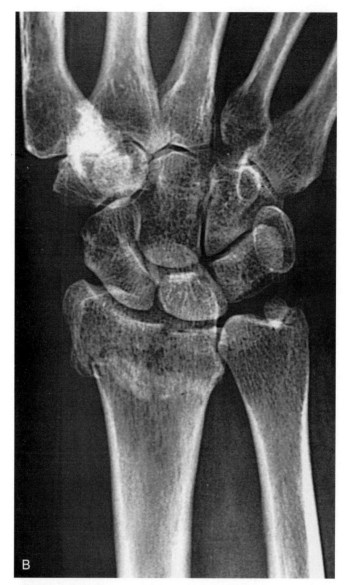

Figure 6-15 *Continued*

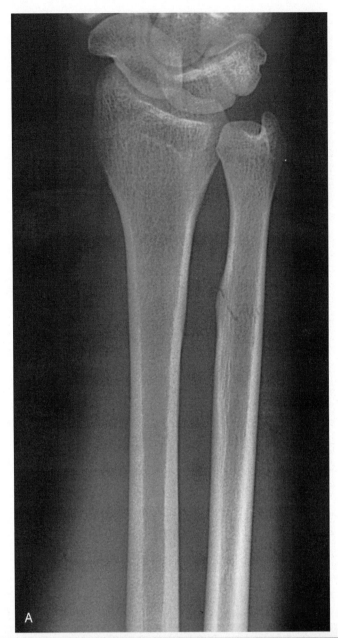

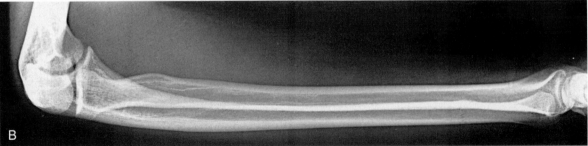

Figure 6–16
Nightstick fracture, (A) frontal and (B) lateral views. Nondisplaced transverse fracture of the distal ulna.

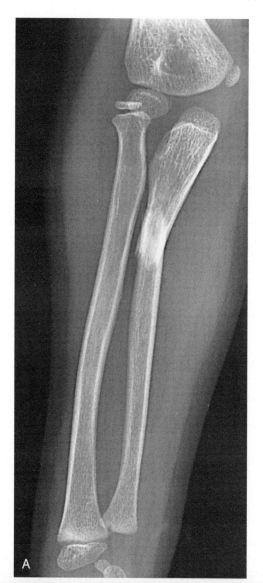

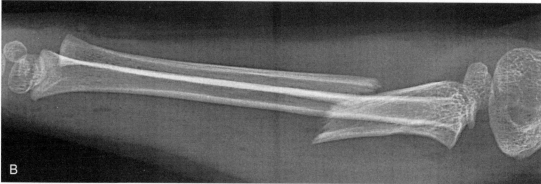

Figure 6–17
Monteggia's fracture, (A) frontal and (B) lateral views. Fracture of the proximal ulna with dislocation of radial head. Radial head does not line up with the capitellum.

WRIST

The wrist has a remarkable range of motion—flexion and extension and radial and ulnar deviation—owing to the several articulations of the radius, ulna, and metacarpal and carpal bones. The proximal row of carpal bones (scaphoid, lunate, and triquetrum) is responsible for flexion and extension. The distal row (hamate, capitate, trapezoid, and trapezium) flexes and extends and, with ulnar and radial deviation, rotates. Force transmitted from the hand to the forearm is often concentrated in the capitate and lunate bones.

Wrist ligament anatomy is intricate (Fig. 6–18). The largest volar ligament, the volar radiotriquetral ligament, extends from the volar aspect of the radiostyloid process across the lunate and inserts on the triquetrum. This ligament acts as a sling for the volar aspect of the lunate. The dorsal ligaments are weaker than their volar counterparts. The scapholunate and the lunotriquetral ligaments stabilize the proximal carpal row. The capitate and lunate bones have no strong ligamentous connection to the radius or metacarpals. The articulation of the lunate and capitate is stabilized by the integrity of the scaphoid and triquetrum ligaments to the capitate. The absence of ligaments between the lunate and capitate allows for a space called the "space of Poirier." With wrist extension, the space of Poirier is filled with synovial outpouching and is an inherently weak link between the proximal and distal carpal rows.

Carpal dislocations are manifestations of damage to various ligaments. Specific injuries are often given names that describe the damage apparent on radiographs (e.g., lunate dislocation, perilunate dislocation, scapholunate dislocation). The exact nature of any given injury, however, depends on the exact magnitude and vector of a force and the position of the hand and wrist at the time of injury. A fall on an outstretched wrist often impacts on the thenar eminence of the hand. This levers the wrist into extension and ulnar deviation. The scapholunate joints tend to be injured first. With greater forces, the capitolunate articulation is lost. With even greater force, the triquetrolunate joint is also damaged, and then the dorsal radiocarpal ligaments rupture and the lunate rotates toward the volar surface. When force is removed, frequently the capitolunate and triquetrolunate dislocations resolve spontaneously. Frequently, the scapholunate space remains wide, and this is evident on radiographs (Fig. 6–19). A worse injury produces persistent capitolunate and triquetrolunate disruptions

(Fig. 6–20), and a lunate (Fig. 6–21) or perilunate (Fig. 6–22) dislocation is seen radiographically.[1]

Scapholunate dislocation is manifested as widening of the articulation between the scaphoid bone and the lunate (sometimes called a "Terry Thomas sign"). Rotary subluxation of the scaphoid is revealed by marked shortening of the scaphoid on an AP or PA view.

A true lateral radiograph of the normal wrist shows the radius, lunate, and capitate articulations as three C-shaped "cups." In a perilunate (see Fig. 6–22) dislocation, the capitate is dislocated dorsally with respect to the lunate (see Fig. 6–22). The hand and the scaphoid are also displaced dorsally. The lunate dislocation (see Fig. 6–21) is a manifestation of dorsal radiocarpal ligament disruption, and the lunate is ejected volarly. It is classic (but unusual) for the capitate to come to rest on the articular surface of the radius. Since perilunate and lunate dislocations are associated with a variety of ligament injuries, it is common for a patient to have some features of both lunate and perilunate dislocation.

The scaphoid bone is exposed to fracture since it bridges the two carpal rows. Most scaphoid fractures occur at the waist of the bone (Fig. 6–23) and tend not to be comminuted. Because the blood supply to the proximal aspect of the scaphoid bone courses through the scaphoid waist, a fracture may be complicated by avascular necrosis of the proximal bone. Scaphoid fractures are often difficult to recognize on radiographs obtained soon after injury. Signs of potential scaphoid fracture include snuffbox tenderness, pain with axial compression of the thumb toward the wrist, and pain with supination of the wrist against resistance.[2] Alternative radiographic approaches to demonstrate scaphoid bone fracture include specific scaphoid views[3, 4] and radionuclide studies.[5] Immobilization of any patient who has clinical evidence of scaphoid fracture is prudent and should continue for 10 to 14 days. At that point, a follow-up radiograph can determine the absence or presence of fracture with great statistical sensitivity.

Hamate fractures can result from direct trauma (Fig. 6–24) or a fall on the wrist. The hook of the hamate may be displaced at the insertion site of the transverse carpal ligaments (Fig. 6–25). The mechanism of this fracture may be interruption of the swing of a golf club, baseball bat, or other object. A carpal tunnel view is helpful in identifying this injury. Pisiform fracture (Fig. 6–26) results from direct trauma. Kienbock's disease may be a complication of a short ulna (ulna minus), and osteonecrosis of the lunate is visible (Fig. 6–27).

Text continued on page 234

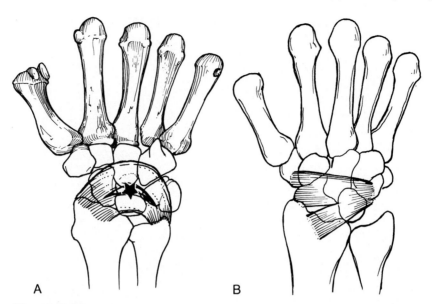

A   B

Figure 6–18
(A) *Volar ligaments form two arches. Star marks the potential weak point (space of Poirir).* (B) *Dorsal ligaments form an arch across the lunate. (Modified from Chin HW, Propp DA, Orban DJ: Forearm and wrist. In Rosen P, Barkin RM (eds): Emergency Medicine: Concepts and Clinical Practice, ed 3, vol 1. St. Louis: CV Mosby, 1992; with permission.)*

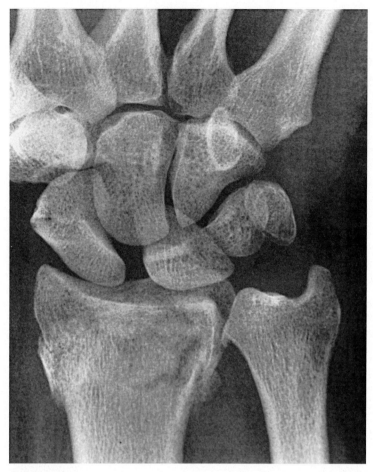

Figure 6–19
Distal radius fracture with widening of the scapholunate space and scapholunate ligament injury.

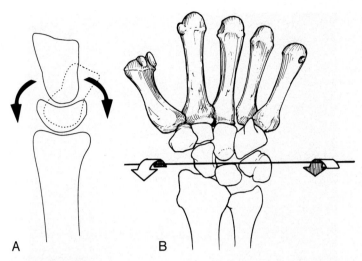

Figure 6–20

(A) *Lateral view. Lunate tilts dorsally if the connection to the scaphoid (dotted) is lost and volarly if triquetrum's is lost.* (B) *Frontal view. Lunate balanced by flexion torque from scaphoid and extension force from triquetrum. (Chin HW, Visotsky J: Ligamentous wrist injuries. Emerg Med Clin North Am 1993; 11:717.)*

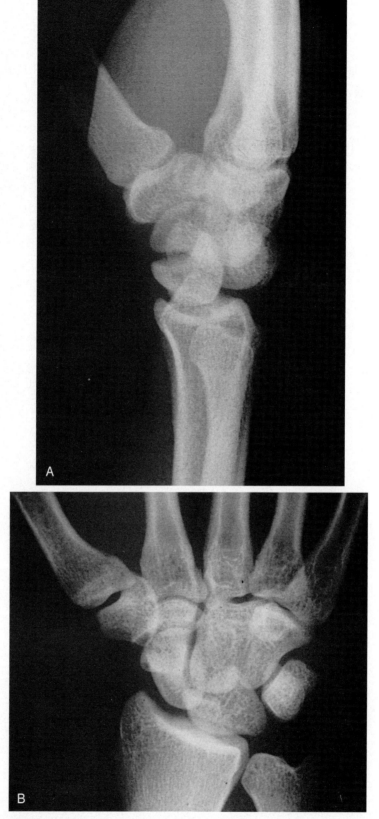

Figure 6–21
*Lunate dislocation. (A) Lateral view reveals lunate to be tipped for-
ward, and the lunate-capitate articulation is no longer present. (B)
AP film reveals a triangular (abnormal) lunate bone.*

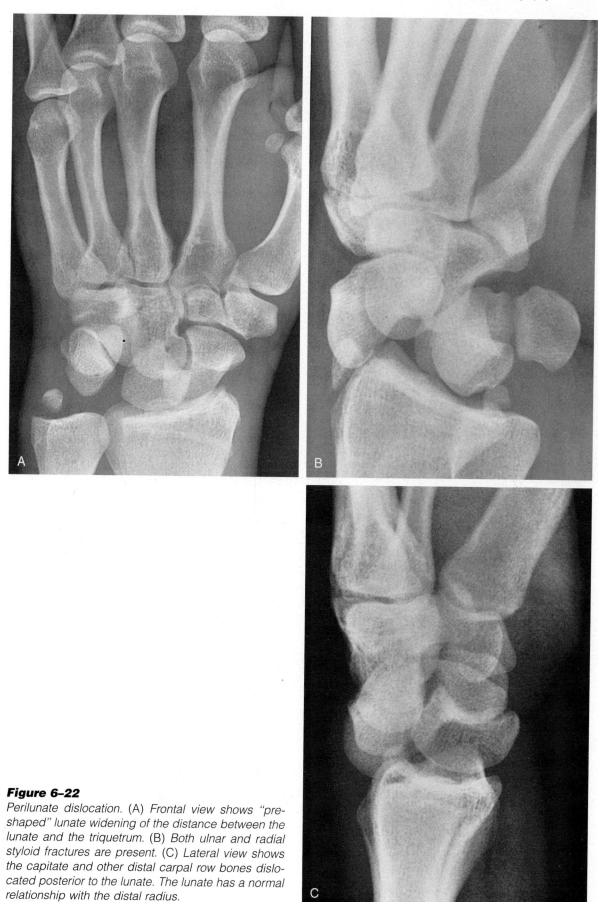

Figure 6–22

Perilunate dislocation. (A) Frontal view shows "pre-shaped" lunate widening of the distance between the lunate and the triquetrum. (B) Both ulnar and radial styloid fractures are present. (C) Lateral view shows the capitate and other distal carpal row bones dislocated posterior to the lunate. The lunate has a normal relationship with the distal radius.

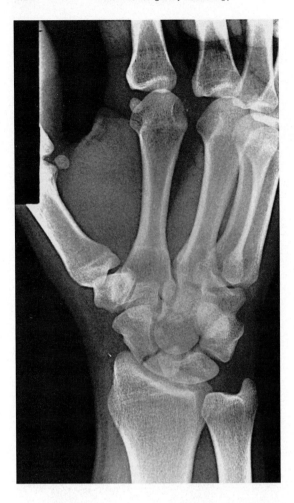

Figure 6–23
Transverse fracture of the proximal pole of the scaphoid.

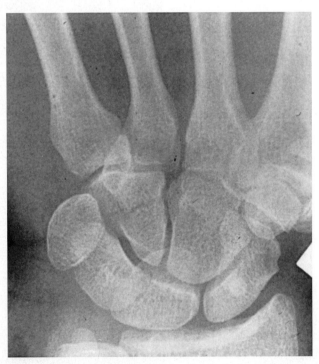

Figure 6–24
Nondisplaced hamate fracture.

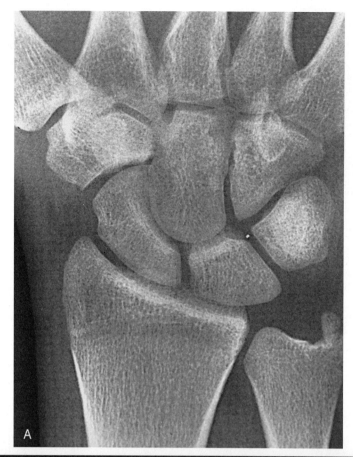

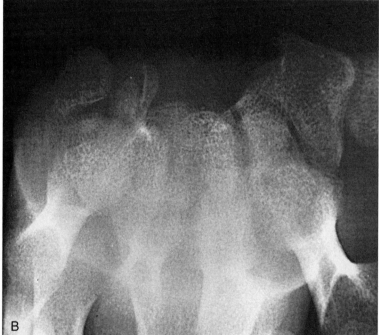

Figure 6–25

Hook of the hamate fracture. (A) Frontal and (B) carpal tunnel views show sclerotic margins of the fracture compatible with an old injury.

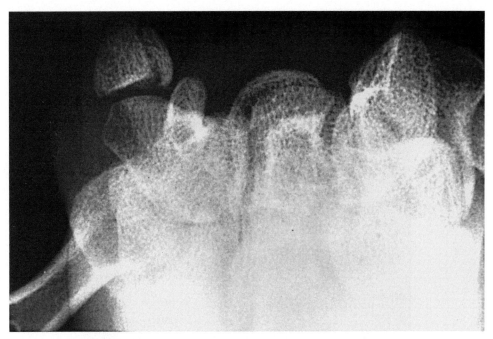

Figure 6–26
Pisiform fracture. Carpal tunnel view shows fracture of the pisiform bone.

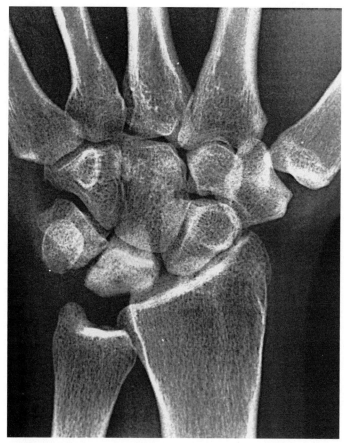

Figure 6–27
Kienböck's disease. Osteonecrosis of the lunate with increased density of the lunate and flattening of its proximal articular surface.

HAND

Hand and finger trauma can appear as both bone and ligament injuries on plain radiographs. In general, these injuries arouse much suspicion on physical examination alone. Radiographs provide details to confirm the clinical suspicion. Routine plain radiographs include AP, lateral, and oblique views. The radiology dictum *one view is no view* very definitely applies to hand injuries.

Phalanges can fracture from direct force or suffer fracture-dislocation from axial or lateral stretch. A distal phalanx can have avulsion fragments from force that is approximately perpendicular to the axis of the finger. A dorsal force may cause avulsion of the extensor tendon and its insertion site, causing a "mallet fracture." Volar and lateral avulsion fractures are also common from joint capsule or other ligamentous insertion sites and from flexor tendons (Fig. 6–28). Axial force often causes dislocation of the proximal (Fig. 6–29) or distal interphalangeal joint or, less often, the metacarpophalangeal joint (Figs. 6–30, 6–31).

Metacarpal fractures are common when an axial force is applied to a metacarpal in a closed fist (Figs. 6–32, 6–33). Fracture of the metacarpal neck of the fifth digit (boxer's fracture) is the most common metacarpal fracture. Such fractures often have rotational deformities that require attention when the fracture fragment is being immobilized. The proximal aspects of metacarpals are also susceptible to fracture and may be less obvious on a quick review of the radiographs.

The thumb has a great range of motion to allow it to be opposed to each finger. It is thus predisposed to certain patterns of injury. The thumb metacarpophalangeal joint is exposed to injury when an object is grasped. One such lesion is rupture of the ulnar collateral ligament (gamekeeper's thumb). Avulsions at the insertion of the ulnar collateral ligament are common on both the metacarpal and the proximal phalanx.

The proximal aspect of the thumb metacarpal may fracture with axial loading. "Bennett's fracture" (Fig. 6–34) describes subluxation of the metacarpal shaft by the adductor pollicis muscle and an anterior fragment that remains attached to the trapezium by its ligament. A comminuted fracture (Rolando's fracture; Fig. 6–35) is a T- or Y- shaped fracture in three pieces.

Text continued on page 242

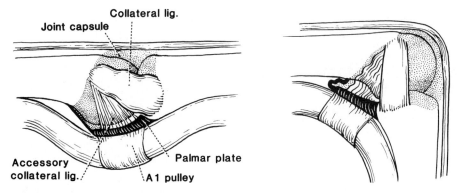

Figure 6–28
*The ligamentous establishers of the metacarpophalangeal joint: the collateral liga-
ment, accessory collateral ligament, palmar plate, and A1 pulley. (© 1992 Kleinert,
Kutz and Associates Hand Care Center; with permission.)*

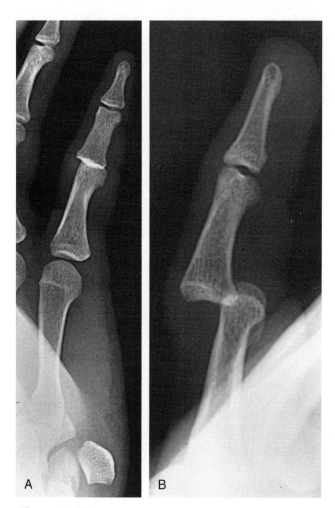

Figure 6–29
(A) *Oblique and* (B) *lateral views demonstrate dislocation
of the proximal interphalangeal joint.*

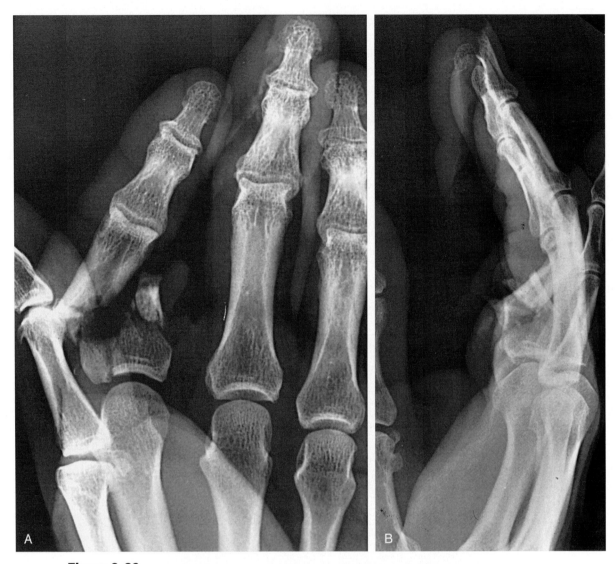

Figure 6–30
(A) *Frontal view of open comminuted intraarticular fracture of the base of the proximal phalanx of the second digit. Marked displacement and angulation are present.* (B) *Lateral radiograph also shows fracture of the distal phalanx of the third digit.*

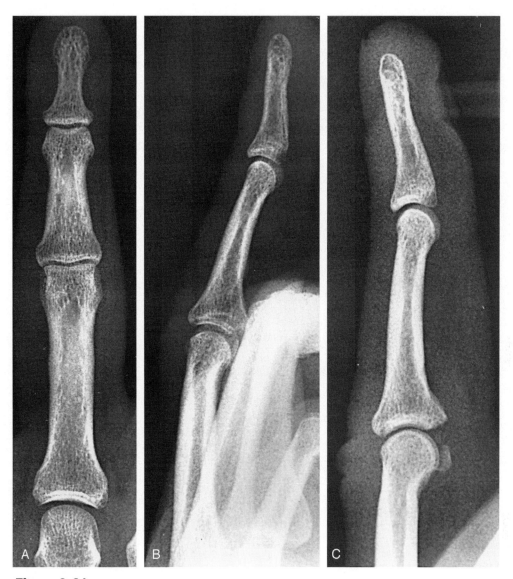

Figure 6–31

Avulsion fracture of the base of the middle phalanx on the volar aspect. (A) Initial frontal and (B) lateral radiographs fail to show the fracture; however, repeat positioning without overlying digits (C) shows it.

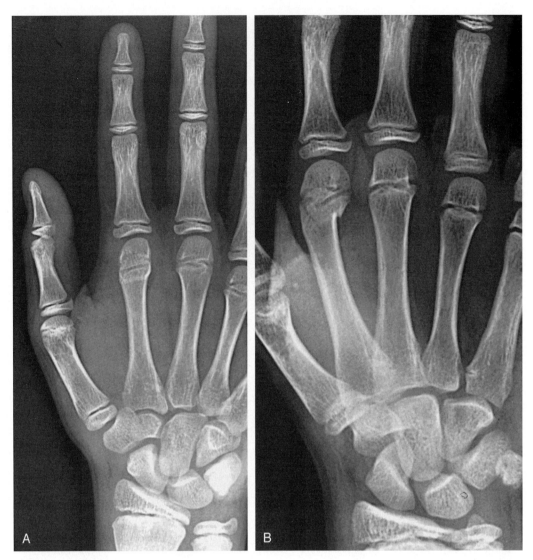

Figure 6–32
Transverse fracture of the metaphysis of the second metacarpal. This is not easily seen on frontal view (A) *but is easily identified on an oblique view* (B).

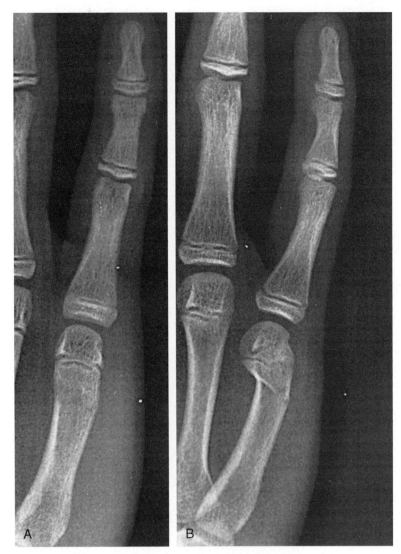

Figure 6–33
Boxer's fracture—fracture of the metacarpal neck of the fifth digit with
volar angulation. (A) Frontal view does not clearly demonstrate the lesion,
but it is easily seen on an oblique view (B).

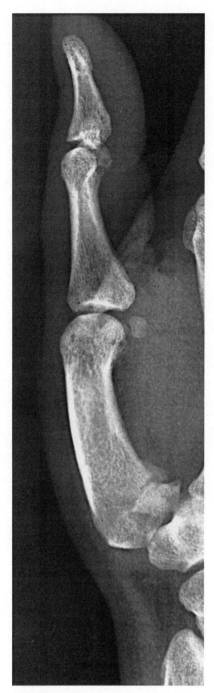

Figure 6–34
Bennett's fracture. Intraarticular fracture of the base of the metacarpal of the thumb.

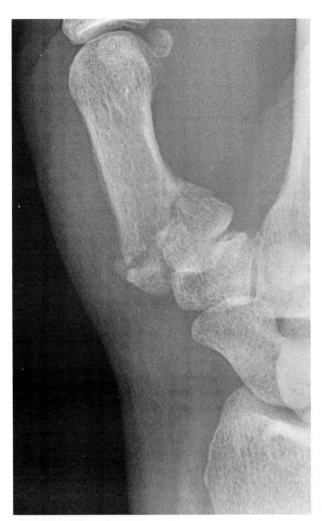

Figure 6–35
Rolando's fracture—comminuted intraarticular fracture at the base of the thumb metacarpal.

REFERENCES

1. Mayfield JK: Wrist ligamentous anatomy and pathogenesis of carpal instability. Orthop Clin North Am 1984;15(2):209–216.

2. Waeckerle JF: A prospective study identifying the sensitivity of radiographic findings and the efficacy of clinical findings in carpal navicular fractures. Ann Emerg Med 1987;16(7):733–737.

3. Roolker W, Tiel van Buul MMC, et al: Carpal box radiography in suspected scaphoid fracture. J Bone Joint Surg 1996; 78B(4):535–539.

4. Roolker L, Tiel van Buul MMC, et al: The value of additional carpal box radiographs in suspected scaphoid fracture. Invest Radiol 1997;32(3):149–153.

5. Tiel van Buul MMC, Broekhuizen TH, et al: Choosing a strategy for the diagnostic management of suspected scaphoid fracture: A cost-effectiveness analysis. J Nuclear Med 1995;36(1):45–48.

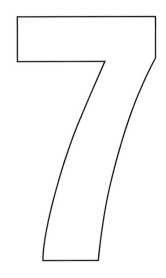

Pediatric Radiography

GARY A. JOHNSON, MD

Normal musculoskeletal development of children leads to peculiar patterns of bone disease. Ossification may occur at the periosteal surface (intramedullary ossification) or along the length of the bone at a physeal plate (endochondral ossification). Long bones typically have one or two physes. The epiphysis is the area of the bone between the physis and the joint. The metaphysis is a wider section of the bone between the physis and the shaft (the diaphysis). Ossification patterns are often very important to interpreting pediatric radiographs.

Toddler's Fracture

Ambulatory preschoolers may sustain an isolated spiral or oblique fracture of the tibia. Such injuries tend to result from a fall with a twisting injury at the foot. These fractures may be difficult to see on radiographs and may show only a subtle disruption of bone. The toddler's fracture may also be detected later, when radiographs reveal fracture healing or periosteal elevation. Toddler's fractures sometimes raise false suspicion of child abuse.

Salter-Harris Fracture

Salter and others have classified fractures involving an epiphyseal plate (Fig. 7–1). Salter I, a fracture through the physis (epiphyseal plate; Figs. 7–2, 7–3), may be diagnosed clinically from tenderness alone. Salter II is a break through the physis and the metaphysis (Figs. 7–4, 7–5). Salter III fractures affect the epiphysis and physis (Figs. 7–6, 7–7), and Salter IV, epiphysis, physis and metaphysis. Salter V is a compression fracture of the epiphyseal plate. Salter I and V lesions are radiologically occult and Salter V may not become apparent until a growth disturbance develops later.

Text continued on page 254

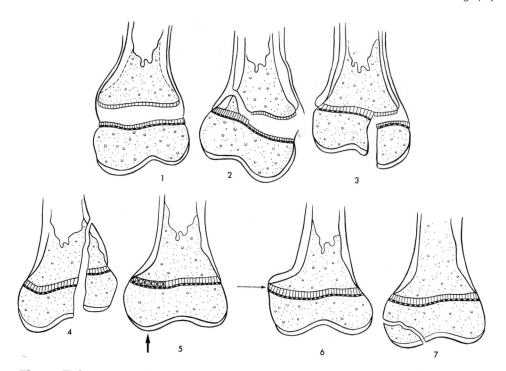

Figure 7–1
Diagrammatic representation of injuries in the region of the growth plate. (From Ozonoff
MB: Pediatric Orthopedic Radiology. Philadelphia: WB Saunders, 1979, with permission.)

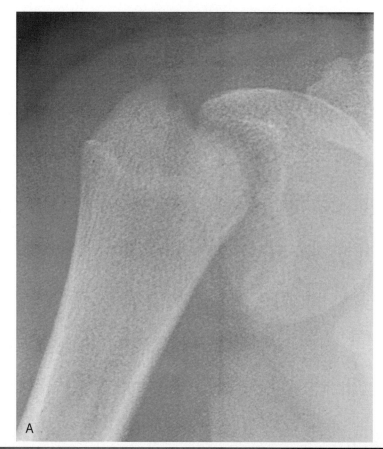

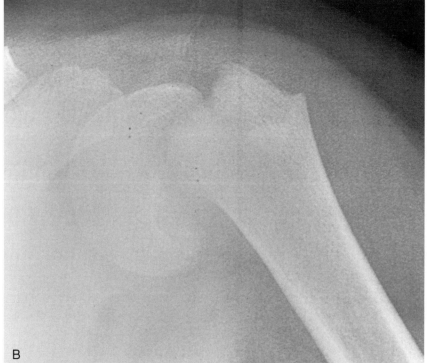

Figure 7–2
Salter I fracture of the proximal humerus, (A) frontal and (B) oblique views.

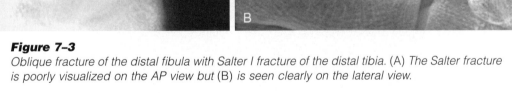

Figure 7–3
Oblique fracture of the distal fibula with Salter I fracture of the distal tibia. (A) The Salter fracture is poorly visualized on the AP view but (B) is seen clearly on the lateral view.

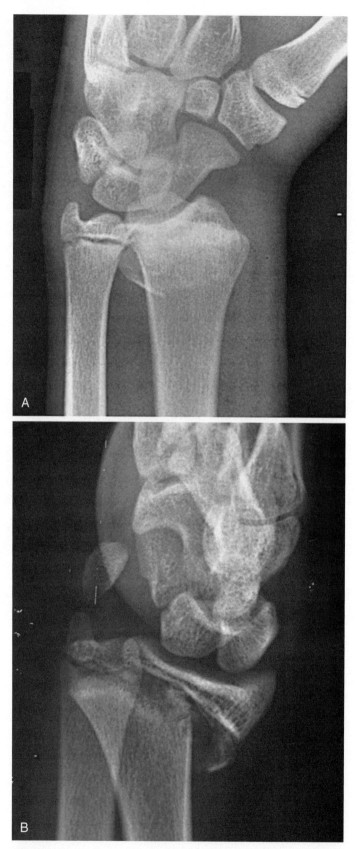

Figure 7–4
*Salter II fracture of the distal radius, (A) frontal and (B) oblique
views. Metaphyseal fracture fragment is attached to the distal
fragment.*

Figure 7–5
Salter II fracture of the tibia, (A) frontal, (B) oblique, and (C) lateral views. Patient has a metaphyseal fracture with widened growth plate.

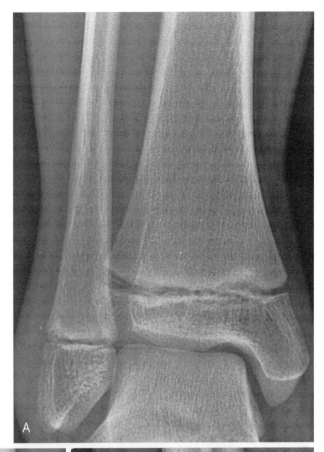

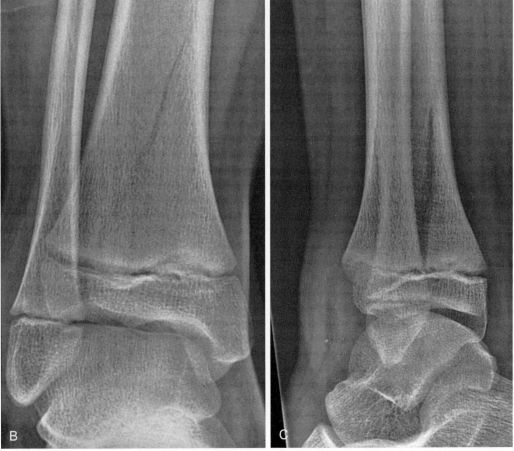

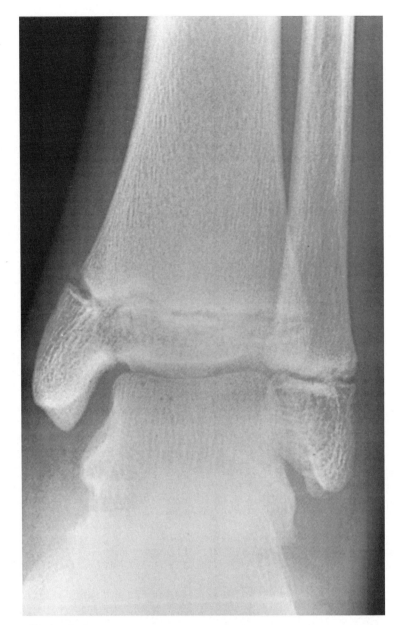

Figure 7–6
Salter III fracture. Vertical fracture line extends through epiphysis, and widening of the growth plate is evident medially.

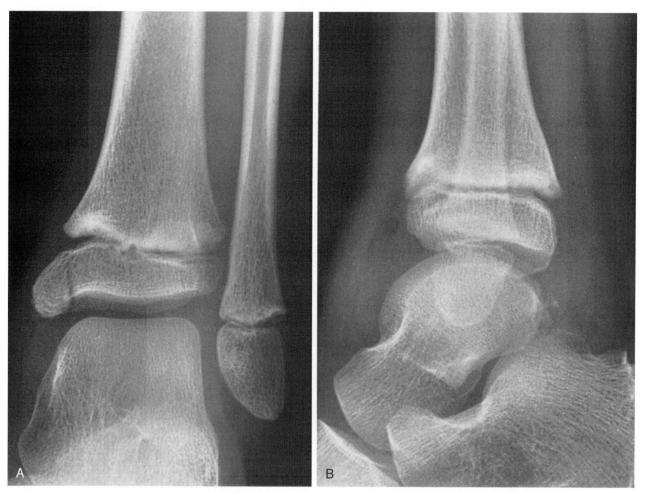

Figure 7-7
(A) *AP view of Salter III fracture of the tibia.* (B) *Lateral radiograph shows joint effusion.*

Greenstick, Torus, and Plastic Fractures

The relative pliability of children's bones may allow a long bone to bend or break in only one cortex (Fig. 7–8). A greenstick fracture (Fig. 7–9) breaks one side of the cortex and bends the other. A torus fracture (Fig. 7–10) buckles the bone without causing a visible disruption of cortex. A bowing deformity (a plastic fracture; Fig. 7–11) of long bones can also occur. On radiographs bowing is demonstrated without any visible fracture line or cortical disruption.

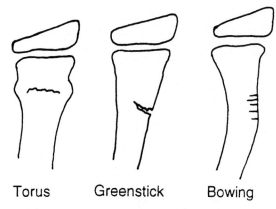

Torus   Greenstick   Bowing

Figure 7–8
Common pediatric fractures. (Wiert PW, Roth PW: Fundamentals of Emergency Radiology. Philadelphia: WB Saunders, 1996.)

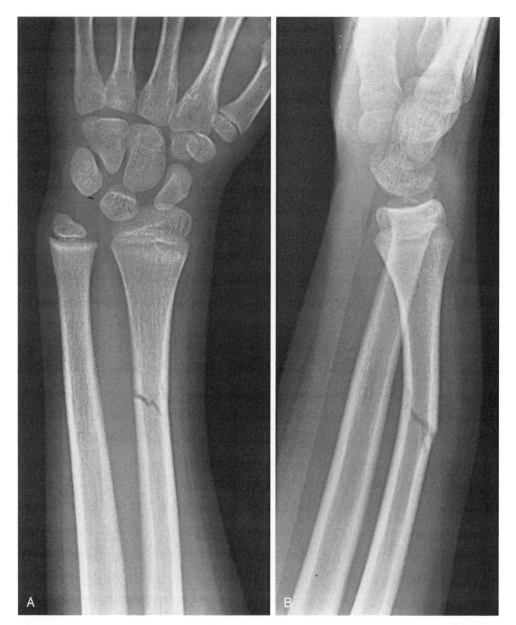

Figure 7–9
Greenstick fracture. (A) *Frontal and* (B) *lateral views show incomplete fracture of the distal radius.*

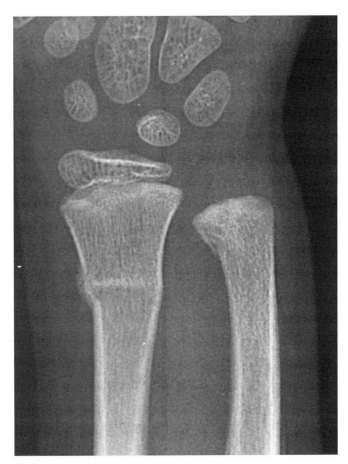

Figure 7–10
Torus fracture of distal radius with minimally displaced distal ulnar fracture.

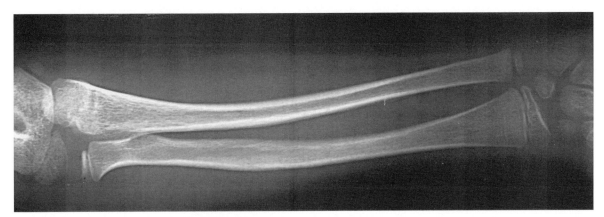

Figure 7–11
Bowing (plastic) deformity of radius and ulna.

Slipped Capital Femoral Epiphysis

Slipped capital femoral epiphysis is associated with obesity and affects children around puberty. The male-female ratio is 8:3. The patient may present with acute or chronic injury. Movement of the femoral epiphysis is noted on AP views. Posterior slips may be better seen on frog-leg oblique views (Fig. 7–12). A line drawn along the femoral neck should intersect the epiphysis. Subtle slips may be diagnosed by comparing the symptomatic and nonsymptomatic limbs. If suspicion of slipped capital femoral epiphysis is strong, AP and frog-leg views should be obtained.

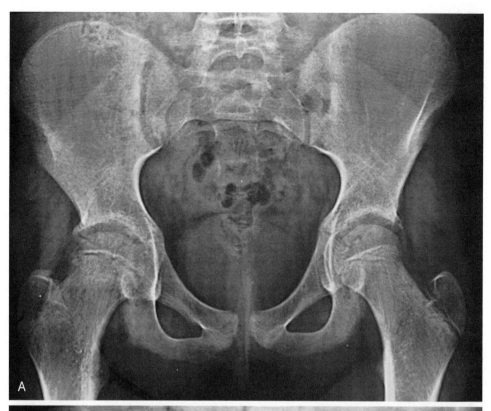

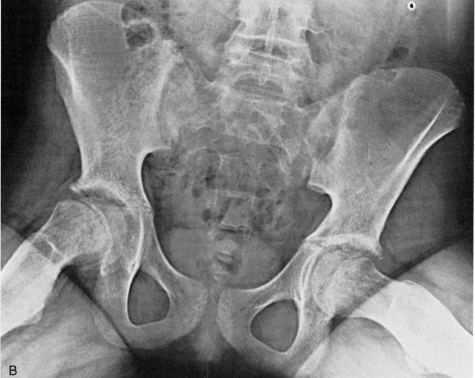

Figure 7–12

(A) *Slipped capital femoral epiphysis on frontal view of pelvis with hips in neutral position shows asymmetry of the hips with slight widening of growth plate on right as compared with the left hip. (B) Frog-leg view demonstrates slippage of right femoral head ossification center.*

Legg-Calvé-Perthes Disease

Legg-Calvé-Perthes disease typically occurs in children of elementary school age. Radiographically, avascular necrosis of the head is seen, and flattening of the humoral head with absorption of bone and sclerosis is apparent (Figs. 7–13, 7–14). Early cases of Legg-Calvé-Perthes disease may show only widening of the joint space from hip effusion. A subchondral line representing a stress fracture may be seen (Caffey's sign). The diagnosis may also be confirmed with radionuclide bone scanning or MRI.

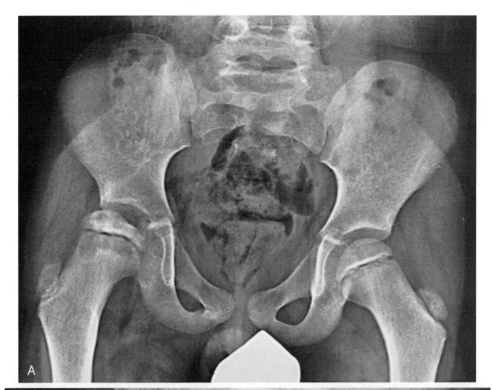

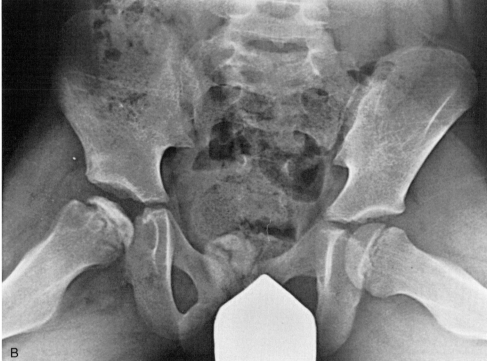

Figure 7–13
Legg-Calvé-Perthes disease, (A) frontal and (B) frog-leg views. Sclerosis and flattening of the right femoral head epiphysis are present, and the epiphysis and metaphysis show cystic changes.

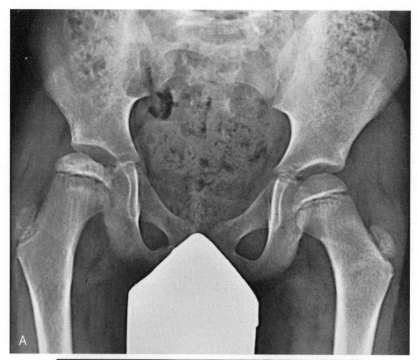

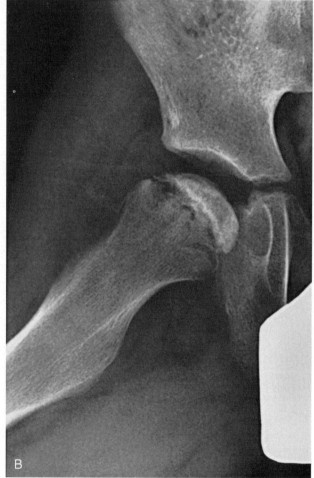

Figure 7–14
Legg-Calvé-Perthes disease. Sclerosis and flattening of the epiphysis of the femoral head are seen on (A) frontal, (B) frog-leg, and (C) Judet's views.

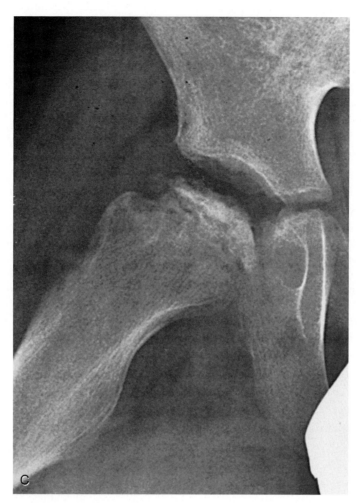

Figure 7–14 *Continued*

Freiberg's Infarction

Freiberg's infarction is flattening of the second metatarsal head (see Fig. 5–53). It is attributed to aseptic necrosis of the metatarsal bone and is more common in girls than in boys (3:1).

Pediatric Elbow

Ossification of the elbow progresses in sequence. The capitellum appears on radiographs between age 3 and 6 months, followed by the radial head. The medial epicondyle appears at 5 to 7 years, and the trochlea and lateral epicondyle between ages 9 and 13. Radiographic interpretation of the elbow depends on identifying the anterior humeral line, the anterior and posterior fat pads, and the radiocapitellar line. The anterior humeral line runs down the anterior aspect of the humerus and should pass through the middle third of the capitellum. The radiocapitellar line passes through the radial shaft and should intersect the capitellum (Fig. 7–15). The posterior fat pad should not be visualized in a normal elbow. When it is visible, a joint effusion is present and a fracture should be suspected. The anterior fat pad may be visible, but in the presence of effusion it is displaced anteriorly to form the sail sign. Visible fat pads may indicate a fracture when no distinct fracture line is visible. Supracondylar fractures are the most common occult fractures of the pediatric elbow (Figs. 7–16, 7–17).

Subluxation of the radial head (nursemaid's elbow) is common after longitudinal traction is applied to the arm of a preschool-aged child. The injury consists of a dislocation of the radial head and disruption of the annular ligament of the radius. Typically, nursemaid's elbow produces no radiographic abnormality.

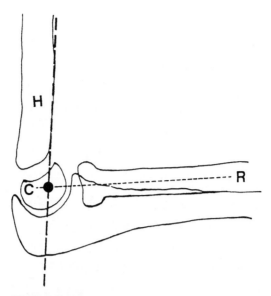

Figure 7–15

Normal anterior humeral and radiocapitellar lines: The anterior humeral line is drawn along the anterior humeral (H) cortex and extends through the capitellum (C) (long dashes). This line normally passes through the middle third of the capitellum. The radiocapitellar line is drawn through the midradial (R) shaft and should normally pass through the capitellum (C) on any radiographic projection (short dashes). (Wiest PW, Roth PW: Fundamentals of Emergency Radiology. Philadelphia: WB Saunders, 1996.)

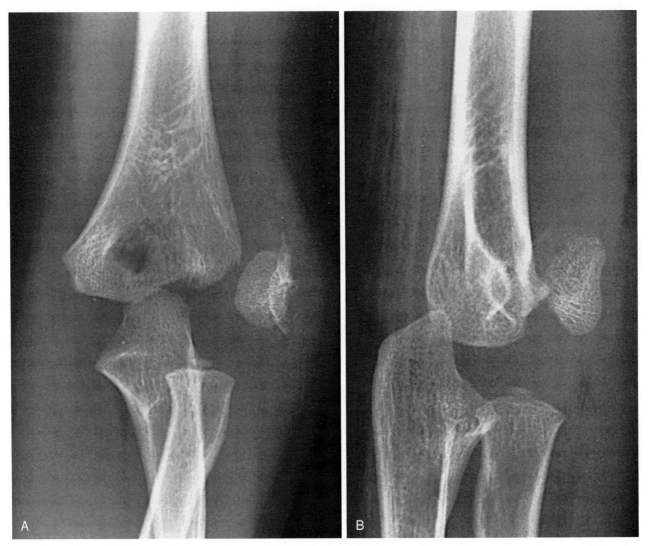

Figure 7–16
Lateral condyle fracture with marked displacement, (A) frontal and (B) lateral views.

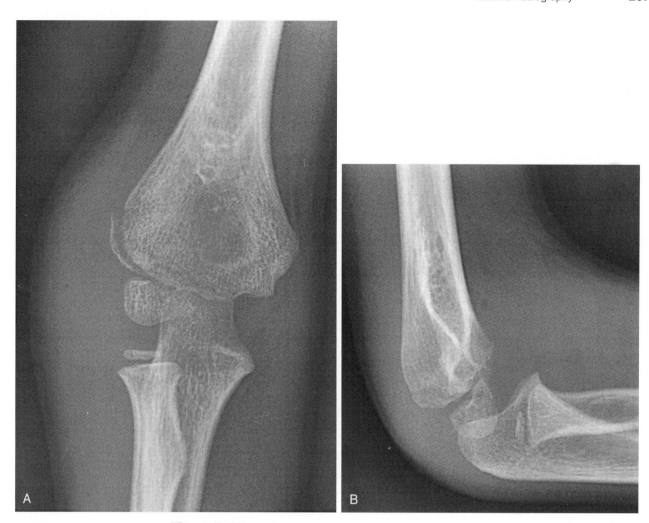

Figure 7–17
(A) *Frontal and* (B) *lateral views of a lateral condylar fracture.*

Osgood-Schlatter's Disease

Repetitive stress on the tibial tuberosity may cause inflammation at the insertion site of the patellar tendon. The tibial tubercle becomes prominent (Fig. 7–18), and soft tissue swelling may be seen on the radiograph. The center of the tibial tubercle physis is often irregular in normal children, and this finding may be mistaken for Osgood-Schlatter's disease.

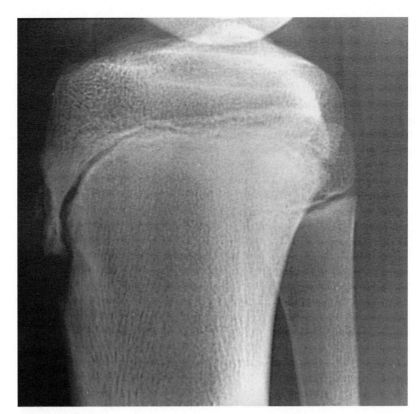

Figure 7-18

Osgood-Schlatter's disease. Irregularity of the anterior tibial tubercle with fragmentation is noted anteriorly.

Child Abuse

Skeletal injuries can result from child abuse or battering. Twisting may create spiral fractures that are very specific for abuse in infants who are not yet walking. Toddlers have, however, been known to sustain spiral fractures from twisting on a planted foot (toddler's fracture; Fig. 7–19). Most spiral fractures of the tibia or femur raise suspicion of child abuse.

Metaphyseal-epiphyseal fractures result from twisting. Chronic avulsion fractures at the joint eventually show striking callus formation. Periosteal elevation often accompanies these fractures.

Direct blows to any long bone may raise suspicion of child abuse. Rib fractures (especially costochondral separations) can be very suggestive of abuse, since abuse is often ongoing. Therefore, fractures of several ages should arouse strong suspicion of abuse.

Radiographic findings may suggest the diagnosis of child abuse, but most often it is identified by combining patient histories and physical examination and radiographic findings. Inconsistent or misleading histories reported by the parent may raise suspicion of abuse. A skeletal survey may be helpful in searching for further evidence of abuse. A radionuclide bone scan can also pick up multiple bone injuries.

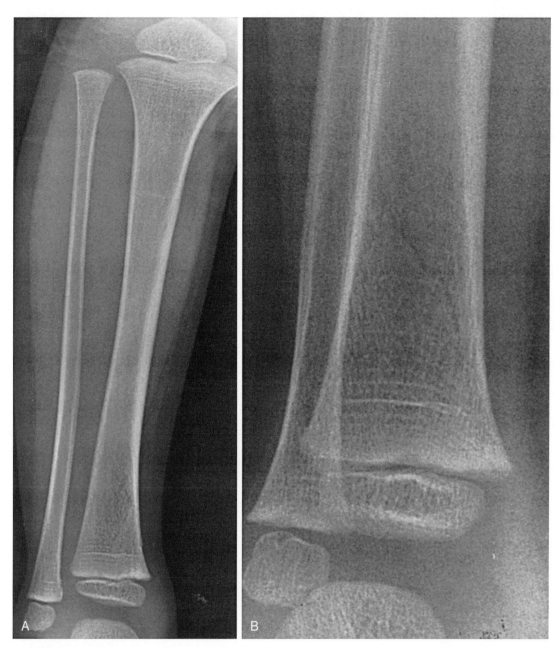

Figure 7–19
Toddler's fracture, (A) frontal and (B) coned-down views. Nondisplaced oblique fracture of the distal tibia extends inferomedially.

Other Diseases

Panner's disease is osteochondritis of the capitellum and appears on radiographs as sclerosis and fissuring (Fig. 7–20). Vitamin D deficiency leads to rickets (Fig. 7–21). Diffuse demineralization is evident, and growth plates are widened.

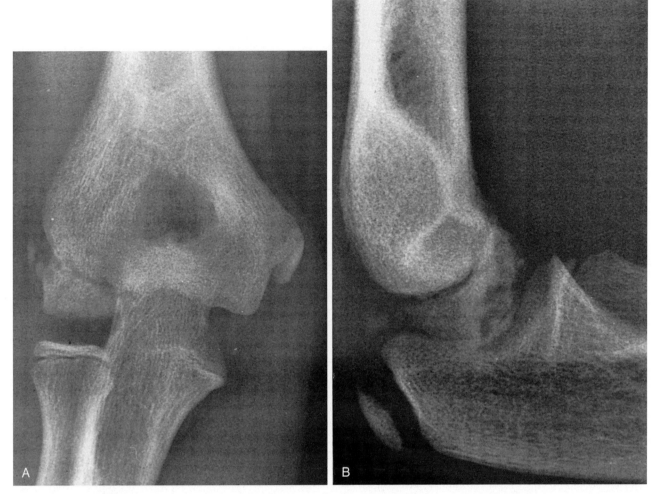

Figure 7–20
Panner's disease. Osteochondrosis of the capitellum with fissuring and fragmentation of the capitellum, (A) frontal and (B) lateral views.

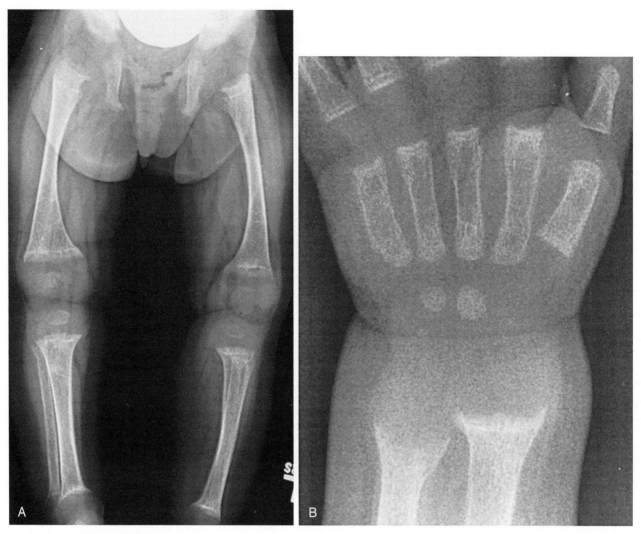

Figure 7–21

Rickets. (A) *Demineralization and irregularity of metaphyses of both lower extremities. Widening of growth plates and cupping of the metaphyses are also present.* (B) *Similar changes also involve the wrist.*

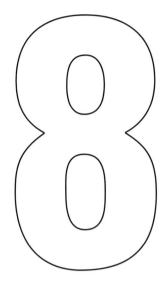

Radiography of Bone Lesions

GARY A. JOHNSON, MD

Emergent films may reveal bone lesions, benign or malignant. Interpretation of a bone lesion must take into consideration that the radiographic appearance reflects both the underlying lesion and its effect on the normal adjacent bone. Factors that should influence radiologic interpretation include location within the involved bone, evidence of tissue changes around the lesion, rate of growth (if known), and clinical factors such as the patient's age and intercurrent medical conditions.

A malignant process may be suspected when there is evidence of bone destruction and inhomogeneous penetration of bone. Proliferation of bone also suggests malignancy, which may have the appearance of a periosteal reaction. In general, a thick, sclerotic rim implies a slow process, whereas a thin shell implies an aggressive process. Intramedullary processes that penetrate the cortex indicate aggressive disease. Multiple lesions may produce a moth-eaten appearance that should alert physicians to the likelihood of an aggressive lesion.

Pathologic fractures are, by definition, secondary to bone disease (Fig. 8–1), either benign or metastatic. Benign lesions include nonossifying fibromas (Fig. 8–2), fibrous cortical defects, osteochondromas, and osteomas. Malignant lesions include metastases, lytic (Fig. 8–3) or blastic (Fig. 8–4) and multiple myeloma (Fig. 8–5). Other abnormal bony processes include intramedullary bone infarcts (Fig. 8–6), which are not radiographically apparent at the time of the infarction but calcify with time and then are visible.

Paget's disease is a result of abnormal and excessive remodeling of bone (Fig. 8–7). Multiple bones are involved, but the pelvis, skull, and spine are most often involved. Areas of both osteolysis and multiple layers of disorganized bone typically are present.

Osteomyelitis may be an acute or a chronic process. Radiographic manifestations include periosteal reaction and osteolysis, but plain radiographs typically look normal for 7 to 14 days after the onset of infection. Bone scan, CT, and MRI may show evidence of acute osteomyelitis 24 hours after onset. Chronic osteomyelitis may occur if bacteria persist in cavities in the bone. A sclerotic margin of dense bone surrounds the cavity.

Brodie's abscess is a solitary lesion. It has a lucent area in the medulla with smooth, rounded margins and a thick sclerotic rim (Fig. 8–8). With chronic osteomyelitis a necrotic piece of bone may persist within the affected cavity (a lesion called a "sequestrum").

Other bone lesions include osteochondroma (Figs. 8–9, 8–10) and eosinophilic granuloma (Fig. 8–11). A "tug" lesion occurs at the insertion of a muscle (Fig. 8–12).

Denervated joints, which lack proprioception and pain sense, may undergo rapidly progressive destruction of cartilage and subchondral bone. Diabetic neuropathy is the most common cause of neuropathic osteoarthropathy (Charcot's joint; Fig. 8–13).

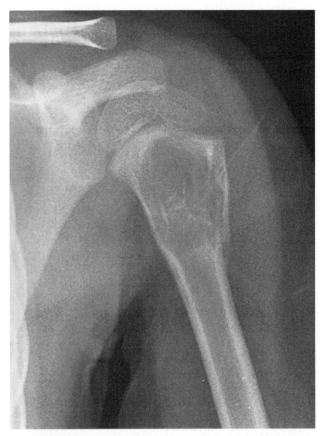

Figure 8–1
Pathologic fracture. Fracture involves a unicameral cyst of the metaphysis of the proximal humerus.

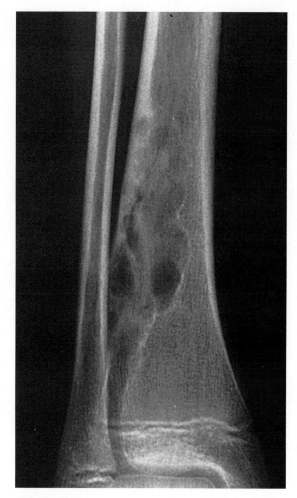

Figure 8–2
Nonossifying fibroma of the distal tibia.

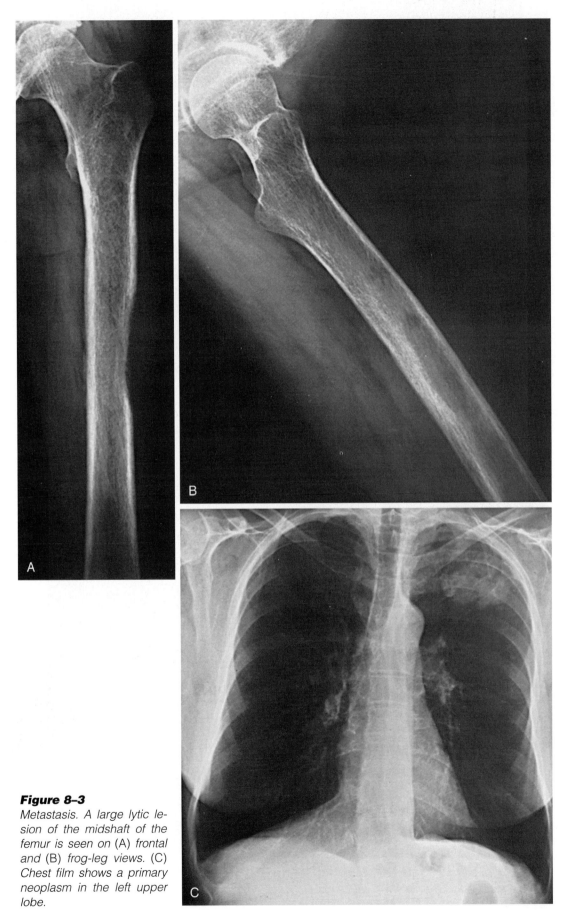

Figure 8–3
Metastasis. A large lytic lesion of the midshaft of the femur is seen on (A) *frontal and* (B) *frog-leg views.* (C) *Chest film shows a primary neoplasm in the left upper lobe.*

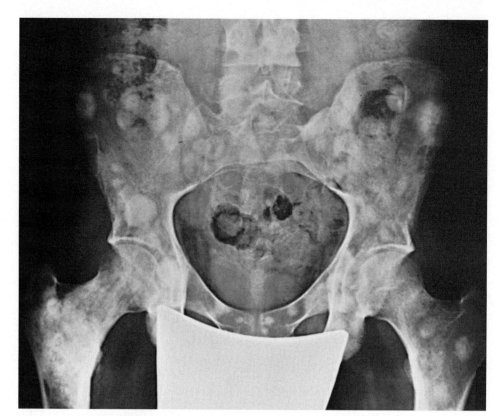

Figure 8–4
Blastic metastases in the pelvis and proximal femurs.

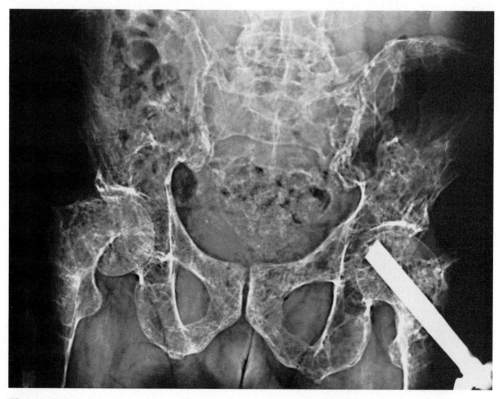

Figure 8–5
Multiple myeloma. Multiple lytic lesions in all bones visualized. Deformity of the right femoral neck is consistent with fracture of uncertain age and fixation device involving left femoral neck and head.

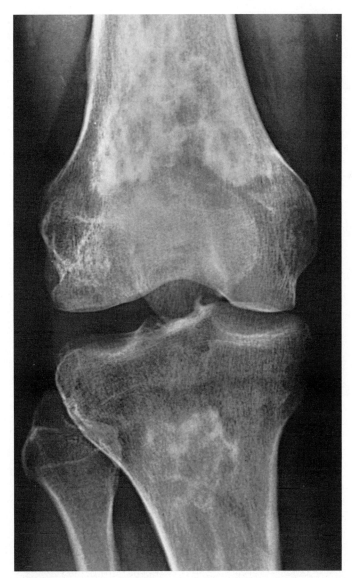

Figure 8–6
Intramedullary bone infarcts. Serpiginous regions of increased sclerosis in the distal femur and proximal tibia are sharply marginated. A small region of sclerosis in the lateral femoral condyle also is likely a bone infarct.

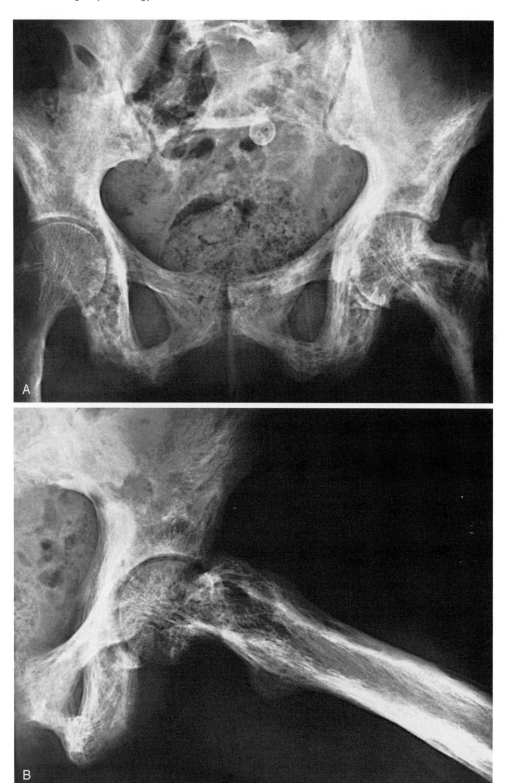

Figure 8–7
Paget's disease. (A, B) Increased density of the pelvis and left femur with cortical thickening and coarsened trabeculae.

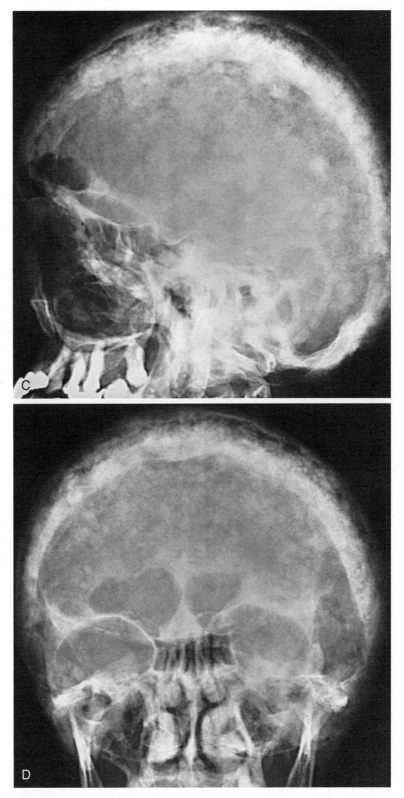

Figure 8–7 *Continued*
(C, D) *The skull shows marked calvarium thickening with "cotton wool" appearance.*

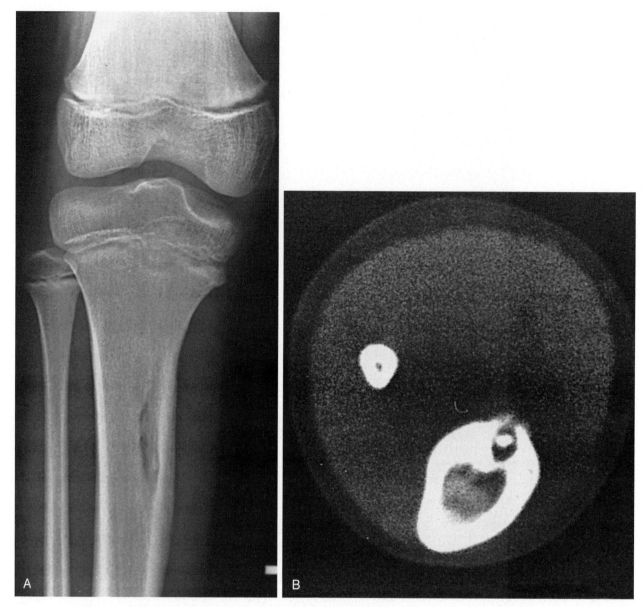

Figure 8–8
Brodie's abscess with sequestrum (a necrotic piece of bone) seen on (A) plain radiograph and (B) CT.

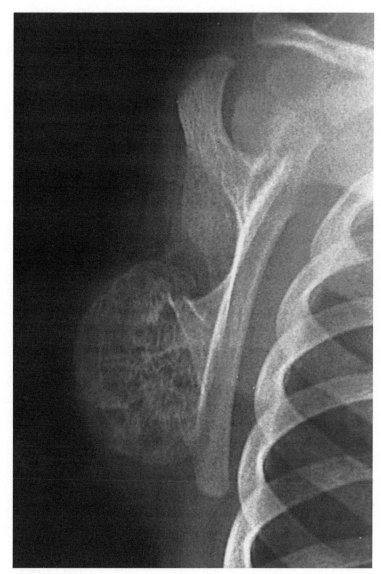

Figure 8–9
Osteochondroma. Large bone exostosis arising from posterior surface of scapula.

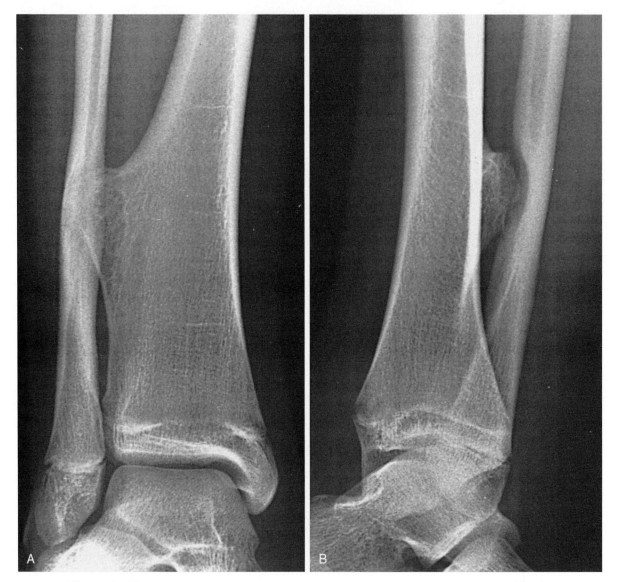

Figure 8–10
Sessile osteochondroma caused scalloping of the adjacent fibula on (A) frontal and (B) oblique views.

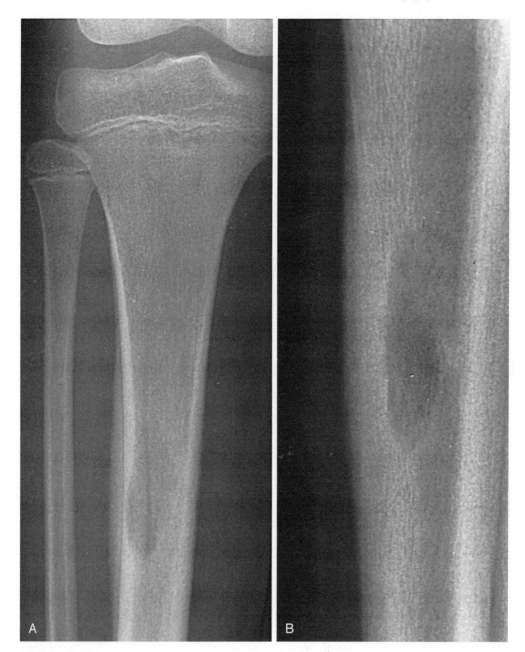

Figure 8–11
Eosinophilic granuloma. A lytic lesion with adjacent periosteal reaction of the midshaft of the tibia seen on (A) *frontal and* (B) *coned-down views.*

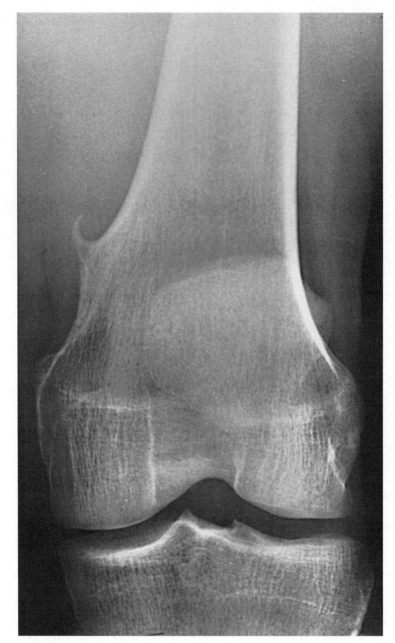

Figure 8–12
"Tug" lesion. Benign bone formation on the medial aspect of the distal femur related to the insertion site of the adductor magnus muscle.

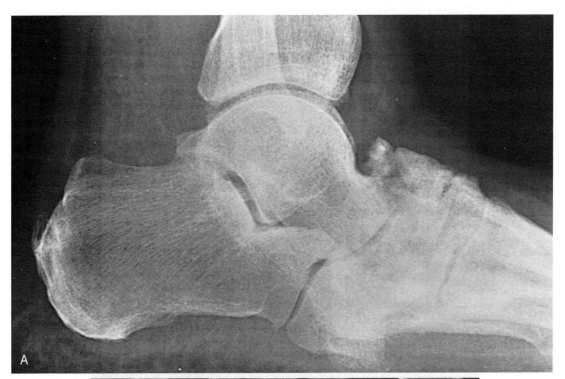

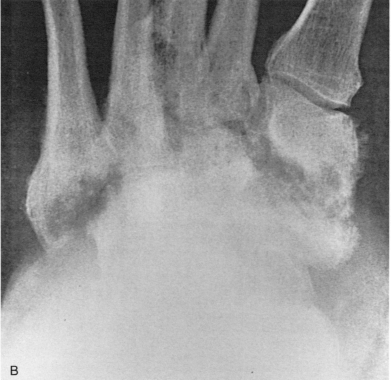

Figure 8–13
Charcot joint. Diffuse joint destruction in the denervated foot of a diabetic patient.

Index

Abdomen, radiographic imaging of, 53–82
  clinical indications for, 56–67
  foreign bodies in, 76–81
  plain, 55
  pneumoperitoneum in, 72–75
  radiopaque structures in, 68–71
  soft tissues in, 82
  utility of, 54
  trauma to, blunt, 34, 44–45
Abdominal aortic aneurysm, 10, 15
Abdominal situs inversus, 16, 17
Abdominal situs solitus, 17
Abscess, Brodie's, 276, 284
  retropharyngeal, 98
Abuse, child, 270–271
Acetabulum, radiography of, 144–147
Acromioclavicular joint, injury to, 202, 204
  spurring of, 210
Adenopathy, hilar, 49
Adynamic ileus, 56, 59
Alveolar edema, 4, 6–7
Aneurysm(s), 10–15
  abdominal aortic, 10, 15
  thoracic aortic, 10, 11–13
  thoracic dissecting, 10, 14
Ankle, fractures of, 172–179
  radiography of, 172–179
Ankylosing spondylitis, 128, 133
Aorta, abdominal, aneurysm of, 10, 15
  thoracic, aneurysm of, 10, 11–13
  trauma to, 16
Arthritis, of glenohumeral joint, 202, 210
Atelectasis, lung, 25
Atlantooccipital dislocation, 108
Avascular necrosis, of femoral head, 148, 156
Avulsion fracture, of fifth metatarsal, 180, 189
  of middle phalanx base, 234, 237
  of posterior tibial plateau, 158, 165
Azygous lobe, 50

Bennett's fracture, 234, 240
Bezoar, 57
Biliary calculi, 68
Bimalleolar fracture, 175, 178
Blood vessels, aneurysms of, 10–15
  trauma to, 16
Boehler's angle, 180, 182
Bone, fractures of. See *Fracture(s)*.
  lesions of, 275–289
Bowel, small, obstruction of, 56, 57–63
Bowing fractures, 254, 255, 257
Boxer's fracture, 234, 239
Brodie's abscess, 276, 284
Bronchiolitis, 18, 21
Burst fracture, of thoracolumbar spine, 128, 130

Calcaneus, bone spur of, 180, 187
  fractures of, 180, 183–185
  in adolescent, normal variation of, 186
Calcification(s), gallbladder, 82
  gallbladder wall, 68, 69
  pancreatic, 68, 71
Calculi, biliary, 68
  renal, 68
Capitellum, osteochondrosis of, 273
Cardiomegaly, 16
  in congestive heart failure, 4, 8–9
Cardiothoracic radiography, 1–50
  anatomic variants in, 48, 50
  heart in, 2, 4–9, 16–17
  lung masses in, 48–50
  pneumonia in, 22–33. See also *Pneumonia*.
  pneumothorax in, 34–39
  pulmonary disease in, 18–21
  pulmonary embolus in, 18–21
  pulmonary trauma in, 34–35, 42–45
  sternal fracture in, 46–47
  vascular system in, 10–16
Cavitary pneumonia, 30
Cecal volvulus, 56, 60–61
Cervical spine, compression fractures of, 108, 118–122

Cervical spine *(Continued)*
  facet dislocations of, 108, 125
  injuries of, 108–127
  radiographic imaging of, 102–127
  spinous process fractures of, 108, 126
  teardrop fractures of, 108, 124
  transverse ligament rupture in, 106–107
Chance's fracture, 128, 132
Charcot's joint, 180, 199, 276, 289
Chest, radiographic imaging of, 2–3
  trauma to, blunt, 34
Child abuse, 270–271
Children, ossification patterns in, 244
  radiography of, 243–274. See also *Pediatric radiography*.
Cholecystitis, emphysematous, 68, 70
Chondrocalcinosis, 168
Clavicular fracture, 202, 205
Colles' fracture, 218, 220–221
Comminuted fracture(s), distal radial, 219
  humeral neck, 202, 206–207
  intertrochanteric, 148, 154
  scapular, 202, 209
  supracondylar, 212, 213
Compression fractures, of cervical spine, 108, 118–122
  of thoracolumbar spine, 128, 129
Condylar fracture, lateral, 266–267
Congestive heart failure, 4, 5–7
Constipation, 56, 63
Contusion, pulmonary, 42, 43
Cuboid bones, fracture of, 185
Cyst, lung, traumatic, 34, 42–44
Cystic fibrosis, 24

Dextrocardia, 16–17
Diabetes mellitus, Charcot joint in, 276, 289
Diaphragm, radiographic imaging of, 2
  rupture of, 34, 44–45
Digits, fracture of, 234, 236–239

Digits *(Continued)*
  radiographic imaging of, 234–241
Dislocation(s), elbow, 212, 217
  facet, of cervical spine, 108, 125
  knee, 158, 168
  lunate, 224, 227–228
  obturator, of hip, 148, 151
  perilunate, 224, 229
  proximal interphalangeal joint, 234, 235
  shoulder, 202, 203

Edema, alveolar, 4, 6–7
  pulmonary, 3–7
Effusion, elbow joint, 212, 214–215
  pleural, 32
  subpulmonic, 32
Elbow, dislocation of, 212, 217
  fractures of, 212, 213, 215–216
  joint effusion in, 212, 214–215
  nursemaid's, 264
  pediatric, 264–267
  radiographic imaging of, 212–217
Embolus, pulmonary, 18–21
Emphysema, orbital, 92
  subcutaneous, 34, 37
Emphysematous cholecystitis, 68, 70
Eosinophilic granuloma, 276, 287
Epiglottitis, 99
Epiphyseal plate fractures, 246–253
Epiphysis, femoral head, in Legg-Calve-
    Perthes disease, 261–263
  slipped capital femoral, 258–259
Esophagus, foreign bodies in, 77, 80–81,
    97
Extremity, lower, radiographic imaging
    of, 158–199. See also specific part,
    e.g., *Knee.*
  upper, radiographic imaging of, 201–
    241. See also specific part, e.g., *El-
    bow.*

Facet dislocations, of cervical spine, 108,
    125
Fat pad sign, in elbow effusion, 212,
    214–216
Femur, head of, avascular necrosis of,
    148, 156
  metastasis to, 276, 279, 280
  neck of, fracture, 148, 152
  Paget's disease of, 276, 282
  transverse fracture of, 148, 157
Fibroma, nonossifying, of tibia, 276, 278
Fibula, fractures of, 158, 170, 172–174
  head of, fracture of, 171
  Salter I fracture of, 249
  sessile osteochondroma of, 276, 286
Fingers, fracture of, 234, 236–239
  radiographic imaging of, 234–241
Foot, radiographic imaging of, 180–199
Forearm, radiography of, 218–223
Foreign bodies, abdominal, 76–81
  esophageal, 77, 80–81, 97
  gastric, 78
  soft tissue, of foot, 180, 198

Fracture(s), acetabular, 144, 146–147
  Bennett's, 234, 240
  bimalleolar, 175, 178
  bowing, 254, 255, 257
  Boxer's, 234, 239
  burst, of thoracolumbar spine, 128,
    129
  calcaneal, 180, 183–185
  Chance's, 128, 132
  clavicular, 202, 205
  Colles', 218, 220–221
  compression, of cervical spine, 108,
    118–122
    of thoracolumbar spine, 128, 129
  femoral neck, 148, 152
  fibular, 158, 170, 172–174
  fibular head, 171
  hamate, 224, 230–231
  hangman's, 108, 116–117
  humeral, 202, 206–208
  iliac wing, comminuted, 136, 138–139
  intertrochanteric, 148, 153
    comminuted, 148, 154
  ischial tuberosity avulsion, 136, 137
  Jefferson's, 108, 110–111
  lateral condylar, 266–267
  LeFort, 90, 96
  Maisonneuve's, 172, 179
  malleolar, 172, 175–178
  mandibular, 90, 94
  metacarpal, of digits, 234, 238–239
    of thumb, 234, 240–241
  metaphyseal-epiphyseal, 270
  metatarsal, 180, 188–192, 195
  midface, 90, 96
  Monteggia's, 218, 223
  nasal bone, 90, 95
  nightstick, 218, 222
  odontoid, 108, 111–114
  olecranon process, 212, 213
  orbital, 90, 92–93
  osteochondral, 180, 181
  patellar, 158–163
  pathologic, 276, 277
  pisiform, 224, 232
  preschoolers', 246
  radial, 219, 226
  radial neck, 212, 216
  Rolando's, 234, 241
  Salter-Harris, 246–253
  scaphoid, 224, 230
  scapular, 202, 209
  Segond's, 158, 164
  skull, 86, 87–89
  Smith's, 218, 219
  spinous process, of cervical spine, 108,
    126
  sternal, 46–47
  stress, of calcaneus, 180, 196
    of third metatarsal, 180, 195
  subtrochanteric, 148, 155
  supracondylar, comminuted, 212, 213
  talar neck, Hawkin's classification of,
    180
  teardrop, 108, 124
  thoracolumbar spinal, 128–132
  tibial plateau, avulsion, 158, 165
    depressed, 158, 166–167
  tibial shaft, 158, 169

Fracture(s) *(Continued)*
  toddler's, 245, 270, 271
  transverse, of femur, 148, 157
  transverse process, 128, 131
  trimalleolar, 176–177
  tripod, 90, 93
  ulnar, 215, 219, 222–223
Fracture-dislocation, Lisfranc's, 180, 193
  of hip, 148, 149–150
Freiberg's infarction, 180, 194

Gallbladder, disease of, radiographic
    imaging of, 82
  wall of, calcification of, 68, 69
Gallstones, 68, 69
Gastric atony, 57
Glenohumeral joint, arthritis of, 202,
    210
Granuloma, eosinophilic, 276, 287
  midlung, 50
Greenstick fractures, 254, 255–256
Growth plate fractures, 246–253

Hamate fractures, 224, 230–231
Hand, radiographic imaging of, 234–241
Hangman's fracture, 108, 116–117
Hawkin's classification, of talar neck
    fractures, 180
Heart, failure of, congestive, 4, 5–7
  radiographic imaging of, 2, 4–9, 16–17
Hematoma, pelvic, 82
  pulmonary, 34, 44
Hemidiaphragm, rupture of, 45
Hernia, hiatal, 56, 67
  inguinal, 56, 66
Hiatal hernia, 56, 67
Hilar adenopathy, 49
Hip, fracture-dislocation of, 148,
    149–150
  obturator dislocation of, 148, 151
  radiographic imaging of, 148–157
Humerus, greater tuberosity of, fracture
    of, 202, 208
  neck of, fracture of, 202, 206–207
  pathologic fracture of, 277
  Salter I fracture of, 248
Hydropneumothorax, 33
Hyperinflation, of lungs, 18, 21

Ileus, paralytic, 56, 59
Iliac wing fracture, comminuted, 136,
    138–139
Infarct(s), intramedullary bone, 276, 281
  lung, 18, 20
Inguinal hernia, 56, 66
Interphalangeal joint, proximal,
    dislocation of, 234, 235
Interstitial infiltrates, in pneumonia, 22,
    23
Intertrochanteric fractures, 148, 153
  comminuted, 148, 154
Intestines, small, obstruction of, 56,
    57–63
Intramedullary bone infarcts, 276, 281

Ischial tuberosity avulsion fracture, 136, 137

Jefferson's fracture, 108, 110–111
Joint(s), acromioclavicular, injury to, 202, 204
  spurring of, 210
  Charcot's, 180, 199, 276, 289
  elbow, effusion in, 212, 214–215
  glenohumeral, arthritis of, 202, 210
  interphalangeal, proximal, dislocation of, 234, 235
  metacarpophalangeal, ligamentous establishers of, 235
Jones' fracture, 180, 188

Kerley lines, in congestive heart failure, 4, 5
Kienbock's disease, 224, 233
Knee, dislocation of, 158, 168
  fractures of, 158–167, 169–171
  radiographic imaging of, 158–171

Laceration, pulmonary, 34, 42, 43
LeFort fractures, 90, 96
Legg-Calvé-Perthes disease, 260–263
Ligaments, of wrist, 224, 225
Lingular pneumonia, 27
Lipohemarthrosis, 166–167
Lisfranc's fracture-dislocation, 180, 193
Lunate, dislocation of, 224, 227–228
  osteonecrosis of, 224, 233
Lung(s). See also Pulmonary entries.
  atelectasis of, 25
  contusion of, 42, 43
  cysts of, traumatic, 34, 42–44
  disease of, 18–21
  hematoma of, 34, 44
  hyperinflation of, 18, 21
  infarcted, 18, 20
  laceration of, 34, 42, 43
  lobe of, azygous, 50
  masses in, 48–40
  neoplasm of, metastasis of, to femur, 276, 279, 280
  radiographic imaging of, 2, 3

Maisonneuve's fracture, 172, 179
Malleolus, fractures of, 172, 175–178
Mandibular fractures, 90, 94
Maxillofacial radiography, 90–99
Mediastinum, air in, 34, 40
Metacarpal fractures, of digits, 234, 238–239
  of thumb, 234, 240–241
Metacarpophalangeal joint, ligamentous establishers of, 235
Metaphyseal-epiphyseal fractures, 270
Metaphyses, demineralization and irregularity of, 274
Metastasis, to femur, 276, 279, 280
  to pelvis, 276, 280

Metatarsal, fifth, fractures of, 180, 188–189, 191
  subluxation of, 190
  fourth, fracture of, 191
  subluxation of, 190
  second, epiphysis of, fracture of, 192
  third, fracture of, 180, 190, 195
Midgut volvulus, 56, 62–63
Monteggia's fracture, 218, 223
Multiple myeloma, 276, 280

Nasal bone fractures, 90, 95
Navicula, fracture of, 190
Necrosis, avascular, of femoral head, 148, 156
Nephrolithiasis, 68
Neuropathic osteoarthropathy, 276, 289
Nightstick fracture, 218, 222
Nursemaid's elbow, 264

Occipitoatlantoaxial region, ligamentous relationships of, 105
Odontoid fractures, 108, 111–114
Olecranon process fracture, 212, 213
Orbital fractures, 90, 92–93
Os odontoideum, 108, 127
Osgood-Schlatter's disease, 268–269
Ossicles, of acetabuli, 144, 145
Ossification, of elbow, 264
Osteoarthropathy, neuropathic, 276, 289
Osteochondral fracture, 180, 181
Osteochondritis dissecans, of talus, 180, 181
Osteochondroma, 276, 285
  sessile, 276, 286
Osteochondrosis, of capitellum, 273
Osteonecrosis, of lunate, 224, 233

Paget's disease, 276, 282–283
Pancreatic calcifications, 68, 71
Pancreatitis, chronic, 68, 71
Panner's disease, 272, 273
Paralytic ileus, 56, 59
Parietal bone fracture, 89
Patellar fractures, 158–163
Pathologic fractures, 276, 277
Pediatric radiography, 243–274
  bowing fractures in, 254, 255, 257
  child abuse in, 270–271
  elbow in, 264–267
  Freiberg's infarction in, 264
  greenstick fractures in, 254, 255–256
  Legg-Calve-Perthes disease in, 260–263
  Osgood-Schlatter's disease in, 268–269
  ossification patterns in, 244
  Panner's disease in, 272, 273
  plastic fractures in, 254, 255, 257
  rickets in, 272, 274
  Salter-Harris fracture in, 246–253
  slipped capital femoral epiphysis in, 258–259
  toddler's fracture in, 245
  torus fractures in, 254, 255, 257

Pellegrini-Stieda disease, 158, 164
Pelvis, blastic metastases to, 276, 280
  hematoma in, 82
  Paget's disease of, 276, 282
  radiographic imaging of, 136–143
Perilunate dislocation, 224, 229
Periosteal reaction, 197
  in eosinophilic granuloma, 276, 287
Phalanx, fracture of, 234, 236–239
Pisiform fracture, 224, 232
Plastic fractures, 254, 255, 257
Pleural effusion, 32
Plicae circulares, 56, 58
Pneumatosis intestinalis, 56, 64–65
Pneumomediastinum, 34, 40
Pneumonia, 22–33
  cavitary, 30
  interstitial infiltrates in, 22, 23
  lingular, 27
  middle lobe, 26
  Pneumocystis carinii, 23
  Staphylococcus aureus, methicillin-resistant, 31
  upper lobe, 28–29
Pneumoperitoneum, 72–75
Pneumothorax, 34–39
  tension, 34, 36
Poirier, space of, 224, 225
Preschoolers' fracture, 245
Pseudotumor, pulmonary, 41
Pubic symphysis, diastasis of, 136, 141, 143
  disruption of, 136, 140
  "openbook" injury of, 136, 141
Pulmonary. See also Lung(s).
Pulmonary edema, 3–7
Pulmonary embolus, 18–21

Radius, bowing deformity of, 257
  distal, fracture of, 219, 226
  greenstick fracture of, 256
  head of, subluxation of, 264
  neck of, fracture of, 212, 216
  Salter II fracture of, 250
  torus fracture of, 257
Rectum, foreign bodies in, 79
Renal calculi, 68
Retropharyngeal abscess, 98
Rickets, 272, 274
Rolando's fracture, 234, 241

Sacroiliac joint, disruption of, 136, 142
Sail sign, in elbow effusion, 212, 214–215
Salter-Harris fracture, 246–253
Sarcoidosis, 49
Scaphoid, proximal pole of, transverse fracture of, 224, 230
Scapholunate ligament injury, 224, 226
Scapula, comminuted fracture of, 202, 209
  osteochondroma of, 276, 285
Segond's fracture, 158, 164
Sessile osteochondroma, 276, 286

Shoulder, arthritis of, 202, 210
　dislocation of, 202, 203
　fractures of, 202, 205–209
　radiographic imaging of, 202–211
　tendinitis of, 202, 211
Sigmoid volvulus, 56
Sinusitis, 90, 91
Skull, Paget's disease of, 276, 283
　radiographic imaging of, 86–89
Slipped capital femoral epiphysis,
　258–259
Small bowel obstruction, 56, 57–63
Smith's fracture, 218, 219
Soft tissues, abdominal, radiographic
　imaging of, 82
Spine, cervical. See *Cervical spine.*
　radiography of, 101–133
　　thoracolumbar, fractures of, 128–132
　　radiography of, 128–133
Spinous process fractures, of cervical
　spine, 108, 126
Spiral fractures, of tibial shaft, 158, 169
Spondylitis, ankylosing, 128, 133
Spondylolisthesis, traumatic, 108
Staphylococcus aureus pneumonia,
　methicillin-resistant, 31
Sternal fracture, 46–47
Stomach, atony of, 57
　foreign bodies in, 78
Stress fracture, of calcaneus, 180, 196
　of third metatarsal, 180, 195
Subcutaneous emphysema, 34, 37
Subluxation, of fifth metatarsal, 190
　of fourth metatarsal, 190
　of radial head, 264
Subpulmonic effusion, 32

Subtrochanteric fracture, 148, 155
Supracondylar fracture, comminuted,
　212, 213
Swischuk's line, 104, 105
Syndesmosis, disruption of, 172, 179

Talus, neck of, fractures of, Hawkin's
　classification of, 180
　osteochondritis dissecans of, 180, 181
Teardrop fractures, 108, 124
Tendinitis, of shoulder, 202, 211
Tension pneumothorax, 34, 36
Thoracic aortic aneurysms, 10, 11–13
Thoracic dissecting aneurysm, 10, 14
Thoracolumbar spine, fractures of,
　128–132
　radiographic imaging of, 128–133
Thumb, fractures of, 234, 240–241
Tibia, eosinophilic granuloma of, 287
　intramedullary bone infarcts in, 276,
　281
　nonossifying fibroma of, 276, 278
　periosteal reaction in, 197
　Salter II fracture of, 251
　Salter III fracture of, 253
　shaft of, fracture of, 158, 169
Tibial plateau fracture, avulsion, 158,
　165
　depressed, 158, 166
Tibial tubercle, in Osgood-Schlatter's
　disease, 268–269
Toddler's fracture, 245, 270, 271
Torus fractures, 254, 255, 257
Trachea, radiographic imaging of, 2

Trauma. See also specific types, e.g.,
　Fracture(s).
　aortic, 16
　pulmonary, 34–45
　　pneumothorax from, 34–39
Traumatic spondylolisthesis, 108
Trimalleolar fracture, 176–177
Tripod fractures, 90, 93
Tubercle, tibial, in Osgood-Schlatter's
　disease, 268–269
Tuberculosis, radiographic imaging of,
　22
"Tug" lesions, 276, 288

Ulna, bowing deformity of, 257
　fracture of, 215, 219, 222–223

Volvulus, cecal, 56, 60–61
　midgut, 56, 62–63
　sigmoid, 56

Wrist, dislocations of, 224, 227–229
　fractures of, 224, 226, 230–232
　ligaments of, 224, 225
　radiographic imaging of, 224–233

Zygomaticomaxillary fractures, 90, 93

ISBN 0-7216-7142-X